PHOTOTHERAPY IN
MENTAL HEALTH

PHOTOTHERAPY IN
MENTAL HEALTH

Edited by

DAVID A. KRAUSS, Ph.D.

Counseling Psychologist
Cuyahoga Valley Community Mental Health Center
Cuyahoga Falls, Ohio

Director
Center for Visual Therapies
Cleveland Heights, Ohio

and

JERRY L. FRYREAR, Ph.D.

Clinical Psychologist and Professor
University of Houston at Clear Lake City
Houston, Texas

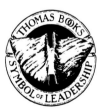

CHARLES C THOMAS • PUBLISHER

Springfield • Illinois • U.S.A.

Published and Distributed Throughout the World by

CHARLES C THOMAS • PUBLISHER

2600 South First Street

Springfield, Illinois, 62717, U.S.A.

© *1983 by* CHARLES C THOMAS • PUBLISHER

ISBN 0-398-04785-5

Library of Congress Catalog Card Number: 82-19403

With THOMAS BOOKS *careful attention is given to all details of manufacturing and design. It is the Publisher's desire to present books that are satisfactory as to their physical qualities and artistic possibilities and appropriate for their particular use.* THOMAS BOOKS *will be true to those laws of quality that assure a good name and good will.*

Printed in the United States of America

CU-R-1

Library of Congress Cataloging in Publication Data

Main entry under title:

Phototherapy in mental health.

  Bibliography: p.
  Includes index.
  1. Photography in psychotherapy. 2. Psychotherapy--Audio-visual aids. 3. Photography in psychiatry. I. Krauss, David A. II. Fryrear, Jerry L. [DNLM: 1. Mental disorders--Therapy. 2. Photography. WM 450.5.P5 P575]
RC489.P56P48   1983   616.89'14   82-19403
ISBN 0-398-04785-5

To Amy, for your support, thorough questioning and profound insight.
To Martha, for your tolerance and help.
To the staff of Cuyahoga Valley Community Mental Health Center for their interest and enthusiasm for this modality; especially Vi Capizzi, Tom Englehart, Anne Gatti, H.W. Johng, Kathleen Miller, Genevieve Polanka and Peggy Reed.
To all people whose interests span a number of areas of human concern, who have more than one perspective on knowing, and who can synthesize their divergent thinking to create new and useful models of understanding.

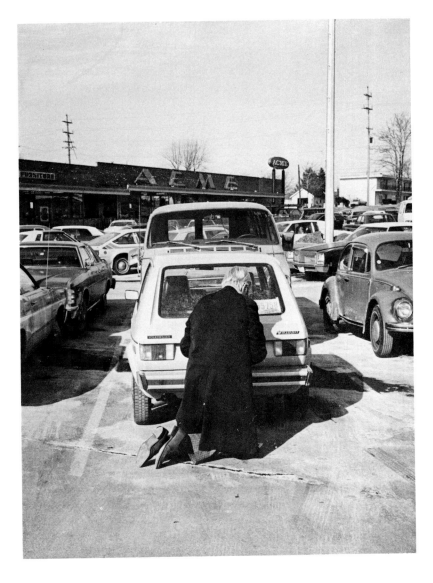

Photo by David A. Krauss.

CONTRIBUTORS

Jeanne Combs is in the Counseling Department, University of Maryland, Baltimore County Campus, Baltimore, Maryland. Her research interests include phototherapy and women and mental health.

Alan D. Entin, Ph.D., is a clinical psychologist in independent practice in Richmond, Virginia, specializing in family psychotherapy. He is a Contributing Editor for *Phototherapy,* the official publication of the International Phototherapy Association, Inc.

Jerry L. Fryrear, Ph.D., is a clinical psychologist and professor at the University of Houston at Clear Lake City, Houston, Texas. He is codirector of the Institute for Psychosocial Applications of Video and Photography at the University and is Managing Editor of *Phototherapy.*

David A. Krauss, Ph.D., is a counseling psychologist at Cuyahoga Valley Community Mental Health Center, Cuyahoga Falls, Ohio. He is codirector of The Center for Visual Therapies in Cleveland Heights, Ohio and is a Contributing Editor for *Phototherapy.*

Douglas Lewis, Ph.D., is associate professor of psychology at Jacksonville University, Jacksonville, Florida. His research interests include attribution of causality and social motivation.

Brett Rorer is a graduate student in social psychology at the University of Florida. His interests include cross-cultural studies and the study of values.

Douglas Stewart, Ed.D., is a psychologist in independent practice in Milwaukee, Wisconsin. He is a Contributing Editor for *Phototherapy.*

Joel Walker, M.D., F.R.C.P. (C), is a psychiatrist who uses photographs as unstructured stimuli with his clients. He has an independent practice in Toronto, Ontario and is a Contributing Editor for *Phototherapy.*

Judy Weiser, Registered Psychologist, M.S. ED., M.S.W., R.S.W., combines private practice with being Director of the PhotoTherapy Centre in Vancouver, British Columbia (Canada). A professional photographer as well, she has special interest/expertise in working with the Deaf, chemical dependencies, and cross-cultural areas. She is also a Contributing Editor for *Phototherapy.*

Ansel L. Woldt, Ed.D., is an Associate Professor of Counseling and Personnel Services Education at Kent State University, Kent, Ohio, and a licensed psychologist in private practice. As a result of being Dr. Krauss's advisor and dissertation chairman, he has experimented considerably with various applications of phototherapy in individual, couples, family and group therapy. His research and training interests focus on gestalt therapy and process variables affecting therapy.

Robert I. Wolf, M.P.S., ATR, is an art therapist and psychoanalyst in independent practice in Forest Hills and Manhattan, New York. He is assistant professor of art therapy and fine art at the College of New Rochelle, New Rochelle, New York.

Brian Zakem, M.A., is a therapist and consultant in independent practice, Chicago, Illinois, completing a Ph.D. in clinical psychology. He is currently Director, International Phototherapy Institute and Founding Editor of *Phototherapy*. His research interests include photo psychodiagnostics and the ways of using still photos, video recordings, and movie film in improving psychotherapy outcomes.

Robert C. Ziller, Ph.D., is professor and Chairman, Department of Psychology, University of Florida.

PREFACE

THE scope of this book is photography in the mental health field, with special emphasis on therapeutic uses, rather than diagnostic ones. This therapeutic use of photography has come to be called *phototherapy* and includes the use of photographs or photographic materials by a trained therapist as an aid in the alleviation of psychological symptoms or to aid in the personal growth of clients.

The purpose of this book is to give an overview of the field of phototherapy, to introduce the reader to the history of photography and therapeutic uses of photography, as well as to show how photography is being used in therapy and what concepts of psychotherapy are most applicable. A pervasive discussion throughout the book will be on visual learning.

The plan of the book is to present original chapters by contemporary leaders in phototherapy. The contributors share an interest and expertise in photography and therapy. Many are both photographers and professional mental health therapists. Several of the chapters are illustrated with photographs taken by the phototherapists or their clients. Mental health professionals from four disciplines are represented among the contributors: clinical psychology, counseling psychology, psychiatry, and art therapy, reflecting the editors' belief that no one profession or theoretical stance represents the only or even the best approach to treatment of emotional or behavioral problems.

Phototherapy in Mental Health can be thought of as a companion to the previously published book by Charles C Thomas, Publisher, *Videotherapy in Mental Health*, edited by Jerry L. Fryrear and Bob Fleshman. Although there are obvious differences in theory and practice between phototherapy and videotherapy, both deal with visual modes of therapy and share many theoretical concepts.

We hope that you will find this book of original essays on phototherapy as fascinating and enlightening as we, and we wish you good reading and good viewing.

David A. Krauss
Cleveland, Ohio

Jerry L. Fryrear
Houston, Texas

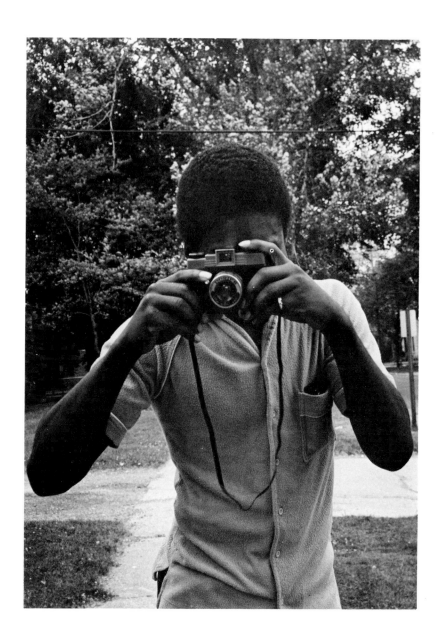

Photo by David A. Krauss.

CONTENTS

PHOTOTHERAPY IN
MENTAL HEALTH

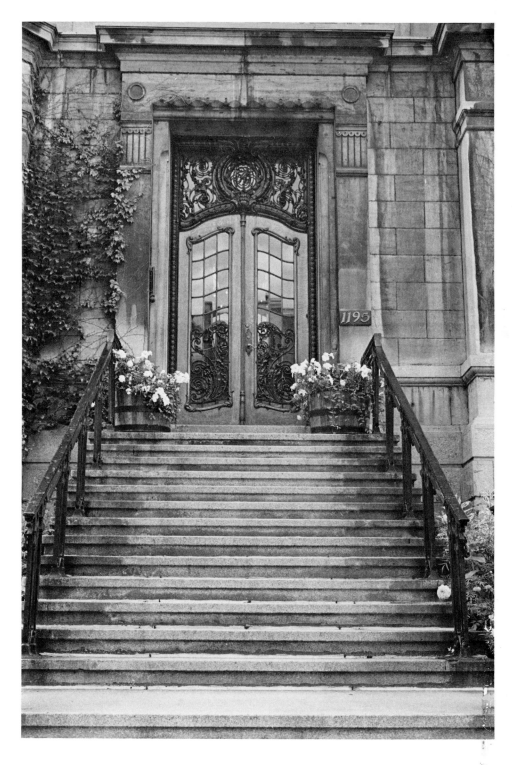

Photo by David A. Krauss

Chapter 1

Phototherapy Introduction and Overview

JERRY L. FRYREAR AND DAVID A. KRAUSS

PHOTOGRAPHY appears to have been invented simultaneously in France and England around 1836. Gilman (1976) states that sixteen years later in 1852 Dr. Hugh Diamond presented a series of photographs of the insane to a London audience. Those portraits apparently represented the first systematic use of photography in psychiatry. Diamond advocated the use of photography as an adjunct to psychiatry, and took photographs of mentally ill clients. He maintained that photographs could be used to study the appearance of the mentally ill, that photographic portraits could change patients' self-concepts, and that photographs could be used as a tool in record keeping so that it would be easier to identify readmissions and patients who needed treatment in the future. His paper on this subject was presented to the Royal Society of Medicine in England in 1856, and can be found along with reproductions of fifty-four photographic plates in Gilman (1976).

Gilman (1982) reports on Kerlin's 1858 use of photography in the Philadelphia Asylum. In Gilman's words, "(Kerlin's photographs) emphasize his charges' ability to return to the world outside the asylum, to be normal as well as to appear normal." Gilman has further documented the use of art and media to show how the stereotypical portrayal of the insane has influenced both societal "perception and treatment of the mentally disturbed," (title page) not only in the United States, but in England, France, and Germany. Auspicious as these beginnings were, it was only in the late 1970s that phototherapy began to truly emerge as a distinct discipline with a rapidly growing body of literature.

Phototherapy has been defined by a number of writers. Stewart (1978) has stated that phototherapy is " . . . the use of photography or photographic materials, under the guidance of a trained therapist, to reduce or relieve painful psychological symptoms and to facilitate psychological growth and therapeutic change" (p. 1). Krauss (1980) has defined phototherapy as "the systematic application of photographic images and/or the photographic process (often in combination with visually referent language and imaging) to create positive change in clients' thoughts, feelings and behaviors."

Fryrear (1980) has divided the literature on the use of photographs in therapy into eleven broad areas: (1) the evocation of emotional states, (2) the elicitation of verbal behavior, (3) modeling, (4) mastery of a skill, (5) facilitation of socialization, (6) creativity/expression, (7) diagnostic adjunct to verbal therapies, (8) a form of nonverbal communication between client and therapist, (9) documentation of change, (10) prolongation of certain experiences and (11) self-confrontation. To these eleven, we add a twelfth broad area, literature regarding phototherapy training.

Each of these twelve areas will be reviewed in some detail, and this introduction will be concluded by a brief preview of the chapters to follow.

THE EVOCATION OF EMOTIONAL STATES

Phototherapy has been used in relaxation training to help clients achieve a state of altered consciousness, relaxation, and/or changes in pulse rate. The use of 16mm film and still slides as aids in audio instruction or in guided imagery have been employed as part of a program of systematic desensitization (Myers, 1977; Vogel, 1977).

Jaffe and Bressler (1980) discuss the nature of the (guided) imagery process and their thoughts regarding its application in obtaining "diagnostic information, for relaxation, to make positive suggestions to alter physical processes, and in the discovery of an inner advisor."

Krauss (1979a) has stated that photographs have the "ability to immediately trigger memories, trigger affect, put the client back into that feeling state, the initial feeling state . . ." (transcription of dialogue regarding the uses of photography in therapy).

Much of the literature relates to the use of photographs to evoke cathartic emotions within verbal psychotherapy sessions. Akeret (1973) described his work with a young woman who had completely repressed a traumatic childhood experience that had been too painful for her to remember. By blocking the memory of the experience, she had been able to deny that it had ever happened, and progress in therapy was slow. By reviewing and discussing photographs from her family album, the young woman was helped to remember the experience and to release the emotions that had been repressed for so many years.

In a study of the response of psychotic patients to photographic self-image experience (Cornelison and Arsenian, 1960) it was found that the presentation of self photographs seemed to induce emotional catharsis in some patients, particularly those patients who destroyed the unflattering pictures of self. It was felt that the patients' act of destroying the unflattering photograph of self might expiate some of the self-destructive feelings, which would leave the individual with less residual anger to control and which would release more energy to cope with reality. The experience of seeing the self in such an unflattering, psychotic state helped to shock the individual into better contact with the realistic self.

THE ELICITATION OF VERBAL BEHAVIOR

The family album method, whereby clients bring into the therapy session photographs of significant others, past and present, has been documented as an excellent method of eliciting verbal behavior. Photographs contain much valuable information regarding relationships and personal values, cultures and ideals (Akeret, 1973). All photographs tell some kind of story and the photograph serves as a visual stimulus for the client to relate his or her own interpretation of what was going on at that frozen moment in time. Entin (1979) has described the use of photographs to get a family to start discussing its process.

Photographs can be used as a visual prompt to help recall memories or experiences that are presently beyond the individual's awareness. Since themes and conflicts of the past also exist in the present, and may carry into the future, it is important to have an understanding of those themes and conflicts in order to cope with them effectively.

Photographs have been employed in life-review therapy by actively encouraging recall of the past (Lewis and Butler, 1974). The aim of therapeutic intervention into the life review is one of guided direction to make it more conscious, more deliberate. Photographs provide a pleasant initiation to interviewing, commenting and reminiscing.

Photographs have been creatively used to engage adolescents into talking about their problems, who had previously been resistant to traditional verbal psychotherapy (Wolf, 1976). The technique was likened to psychodrama or even free association, which puts the individual into close contact with material from the unconscious. The creative use of the photographs allowed concrete form to each of the elements of the patient's unconscious conflicts. The process familiarized the individuals with their own images and unconscious processes.

McKinney (1979) reports on the successful use of photography in psychotherapy with an adolescent. The article states that "the boy was able to discuss many formerly hidden aspects of his self-concept after the photos made it easier for him to focus on and talk about himself."

Weal (1980) reported on a project done by Hogan and Villaneuvas where "normal" and handicapped high school students photographed each other. Five "normal" and four severely orthopedically handicapped young people made photos of each other and discussed them for a ten-session therapy program. Weal reports:

> Hogan found that non-handicapped kids were almost as self-conscious about their appearance as the handicapped kids were. She also found that, as she had hoped, the very act of discussing disabilities openly made the "normal" students more accepting of their disabled peers and more willing to form friendships with them.

Loellbach (1978) describes her work with a client whose somatic complaints were diagnosed as having emotional origins. The use of family photographs allowed the client to review his past and uncover the specific issues of his guilt, anger and his feelings of inadequacy. She concludes, "the photographs provided an interesting and enjoyable means of redirecting Wayne's thoughts outside of his own body. They provided a gentle and nonconfrontive means of cutting through repressions and helping Wayne get in touch with his feelings. They are also providing an on-going support and reinforcement of progress in therapy."

Poli (1979) described Walker's use of photographs with his clients. His personal photographs, which were originally hung in his office for decoration, were found to be useful in eliciting spontaneous client response. Walker (1980) more thoroughly describes his work in this area of using his "purposefully ambiguous and abstract" images in directive and nondirective ways. A number of case illustrations are presented. He concludes, "Both techniques helped effect change by a heightened awareness of how the patient perceives the world. He can potentially learn alternative ways and utilize his adaptive resources to alter his/her perception of this world."

MODELING

Although there is a wealth of literature on the use of videotape and film for modeling purposes, the use of photographs for the modeling of grooming, dress and appropriate behavior is only recently beginning to receive much attention. Particularly intriguing is the notion of one's self as model, or imitating oneself as portrayed on film or videotape.

Several studies have been undertaken whose purpose was to enhance the self-esteem and social behavior of children and juvenile delinquents through a program of self-modeling and self-confrontation (Ammerman and Fryrear, 1975; Fryrear, Nuell and Ridley, 1974; Fryrear, Nuell and White, 1977; Vardell, McClellan and Fryrear, 1982; Milford, Swank and Fryrear, 1980). Individual photographs of the subjects in various postures, exhibiting various grooming skills and engaged in various appropriate social interactions were taken and given back to the subjects as records of their participation. The photographs of the self engaged in these desired behaviors served as realistic and idealistic models for the participants. Photography allowed for the individuals to model the desired activity or behavior and provided a permanent visual record that allowed the individuals to see themselves objectively and accurately.

Titus (1976) discusses a rather unique use of family photographs to provide role rehearsal or modeling of future parenting roles. It was felt that photographs promote the transition to parenthood via modeling and/or ritualization which enhances commitment to the new parenting role. Titus pointed out that role behaviors are observable processes, and that observers of family photos can note observable and repetitive actions of the parenting role to be emulated by offspring.

MASTERY OF A SKILL

As Zakem (1977) has reported, the learning of photography as a skill is one of the goals of the phototherapy program at Ravenswood Hospital Medical Center. Wolf (1978) has also reported on the ego-strengthening effects of mastering the skill of photography with an inner-city youth. The case study revealed a boy whose father and older brother had both died of heroin over-doses, and indicated that the boy was beginning to get involved in illegal activities as well. Although the focus of the study was on the establishment of the therapeutic alliance between the therapist and the boy through the photography program, Wolf reported that the youth was able to see quick results using photography and to feel a sense of accomplishment after learning the technical process and mastering the procedure.

Because there is such a wide range of skills required in learning photography, from simple operation of pocket instamatic cameras, to self-developing cameras, to highly sophisticated printing techniques, people of all range of abilities can be taught to master the requirements. Starrels (1978) reports of a project teaching photography to Headstart youngsters, and of the pleasures these youngsters received from learning to photograph.

Smith (1978) also used Polaroid® cameras to make portraits of children in therapy. She concludes, "The contributions of photographing a child as part of therapy include giving the child a greater sense of power and self-determination, affirming identity, creating a better self image."

Nelson-Gee (1975), in working with a nonverbal young boy, used a Polaroid camera as a method to communicate with him and to teach him life skills. Through photo work and traditional therapist "mirroring," she helped him to expand his vocabulary and to speak in sentences. She also improved his self-concept so that he could see himself as different from objects, such as his lunch box or toys. She concluded that Polaroid photography provides visual and tactile sensation and instant feedback. It also established communication through the common ground of the photograph.

In asking the question, "What do you see?" she provided a framework for the client to say what he saw when he focused on an image. The client learned to focus on one set of stimuli at a time, to abstract information, to understand sequential relationships, and the connection between cause and effect. He also learned to wait for the photograph to develop (a higher tolerance of frustration) and to feel happy and proud of his photographic work as a product. She concludes:

> The Polaroid camera was an especially good therapeutic tool for the work Jay and I did together. Photography provided a means of physically touching this child for whom words had less effect and less meaning than did visual and tactile stimulation. (Nelson-Gee, 1975)

Aronson and Graziano (1976) completed a study in which the mastery of photographic skills by elderly residents of a nursing home was one of the bene-

ficial aspects of a phototherapy project. Of the ten subjects who were interviewed at the conclusion of the study, only seven were able to recall the
photography project. However, all seven participants who recalled the activity
reported that they had enjoyed the activity, had benefitted, and would like the
activity to continue. Experimental results indicated that the photographic experience was associated with significantly increased positive attitude regarding
"older people" and "younger people" (p. 367).

FACILITATION OF SOCIALIZATION

Milgram (1977) stated that photography has become an integral part of
human nature, and that the effects of a camera's presence has effects on the
social behavior of those participating in the photographing procedure. Experimental results have indicated that antisocial behavior has been inhibited in
the camera's presence, and prosocial behavior, such as donating more money
in a camera's presence, has been documented. The habit of taking pictures is
widespread, almost worldwide, and most people are willing to be photographed. Many are curious to see the end product.

The act of taking a picture is a social experience focusing necessarily from
self upon other. In a very real way the "privileged space" between photographer
and subject is violated and, however superficial, an act of relating takes place.
Photography can be used as as aid in meeting people, helping to initiate conversation, and serving as a common interest.

Miller (1962), in an experiment at Louisiana State Mental Hospital,
demonstrated that one could increase social interaction between patients and
between patients and staff by taking random photos, i.e. snapshots, of patients
and displaying them on the walls.

Family therapists have used photographs to encourage openness and sharing by stimulating conversation. The family album is, after all, a visual,
historical record of social interactions and relationships within that family.
Akeret (1973) has used photographs from family albums to uncover the
subtleties and complexities of an individual's relationship with other people to
pinpoint and correct problems in socialization skills.

Titus (1976) reported on the use of family photographs as a role rehearsal,
or as an aid to introduce new parents to the parenting role. Socialization was
aided through the discussion of the common interest, parenting.

Williams and Williams (1981) describe the use of photographs to ease problems of transition from one residential setting to another. The concrete nature
of the photographs allowed the participants (labelled mentally retarded) to
preserve images which were important to them and to show them what their
future surroundings would look like. Results included:

> (1) A sense of accomplishment was developed by taking photographs. (2) The
> photograph album was seen as a valuable possession. (3) The community album made

discussion of group living concrete. (4) Photography helped establish rapport with staff . . . (6) Photography became a common interest in the home. (7) Photography acted as a means of communication . . . (8) Dealing with past close relationships was enhanced.

The use of photography as an aid in meeting people and in initiating conversations has received some attention (Ammerman and Fryrear, 1975; Aronson and Graziano, 1976; Fryrear, Nuell and Ridley, 1974; Fryrear, Nuell and White, 1977; Spire, 1973). When one is engaged in an activity that is social in nature, it is difficult to exclude verbal interaction as well, both in process and outcome.

CREATIVITY/EXPRESSION

Sontag (1973) stated that to collect photographs is to collect the world. Photography has thus far not found full acceptance among artists as an artistic mode, perhaps because industrialization provided social uses for the focus of the camera, or perhaps because photography is recognized as a widely practiced type of amusement, lacking the dignity of "pure art form." But one cannot deny that photography, in the hands of an individual, is a creative expression of that individual.

Wolf (1976) reported on a project that used photographs in combination with art, which allowed the patient to construct and familiarize himself with his own fantasy productions and unconscious processes. The approach proved particularly effective with adolescents who had been previously resistant to treatment.

Turner-Hogan (1981) describes her use of phototherapy in classroom groups to enhance self-esteem of "latency age children" who were experiencing "academic and/or behavior problems." She states that children found the use of equipment inherently interesting and a motivation for fulfilling assignments. Zakem (1977) describes various uses of phototherapy in a day treatment unit of a psychiatric hospital. He states: "The options phototherapy provides allow for the creative integration of phototherapy's parent disciplines — psychotherapy and photography."

Using a phenomenological approach, Tyding (1973) used very basic photography equipment with twenty-five uncommunicative primary grade students. The results showed significantly improved parent-child communication. He states:

> With a camera, children are forced to focus and concentrate upon a single perception. As they become more practiced, they tend to be more painstaking about arranging people and things to their satisfaction. With his world put in order the child begins to use his photos as a surrogate of reality for starting up conversations, which in turn develop into new friendships. Eventually, the child himself becomes a part of his new world discovered through the lens.

Using the same approach Hedges (1972) asked normal elementary school students to photograph whatever they wished. He subsequently let the children discuss the photographs with him (in the role of nondirective facilitator) and discovered that it was a method of opening up their perceptions and changing their self-concepts.

Nicoletti (1972) worked in a similar manner with ninety normal fourth grade boys and girls from a suburban-rural elementary school district. He found significant change in self-concept for both boys and girls in the treatment group as a result of the photo experience.

Hattersley (1971) has suggested that one can creatively use photography to discover who one is — that is to use the medium as a path to awareness. He suggests exercises to "unearth your unconscious psychic symbols and to discover what they really mean to you — to help you overcome cultural and self-conditioning — to help you understand your family better — etc." (p.9). Hattersley (1980) summarized his thinking, "In this short essay I've attempted to tell you some of the reasons why photography is good for you. You shouldn't be surprised that this is so, because creativity as such has long been considered as healthful. In creating things we also create ourselves." White (1962, 1969) has also discussed the creative and expressive aspects of photography toward self-understanding.

McDougall-Treacy (1979) conducted photography self-awareness workshops to give people data about their own unique ways of viewing and valuing, as well as to provide them with new ways of expressing themselves via the camera. Indeed, she spoke of the person as the camera experience. Levinson (1979) also sees the photographic experience as an expression of that person's inner world, a world which even that individual rarely has an opportunity to glimpse. He pointed out the ambiguity and expressiveness inherent in photography and compared each picture-taking assignment to a type of projective technique, and followed the assumption that pictures more closely represent inner mental life than words.

DIAGNOSTIC ADJUNCT TO VERBAL THERAPIES

Akeret (1973) alluded to the use of photographs and of the family album as an aid to the interpretation of the unconscious meanings of gestures, postures and expressions of those photographed. He proposed that his technique of analyzing photographs, photoanalysis, would allow individuals to discover what the people who were photographed really think about themselves and each other. Photoanalysis is achieved through analysis of the kinds of pictures taken, the poses, distancing and body language of those photographed and by the poses not selected to be shared with the therapist. Furthermore, photographs can show specific times when dramatic changes take place in a client's life. Photos can be used as a scale against which clients' perceptions and relationships can be measured by others.

Graham (1967) described the use of photographs in a research project in which Polaroid photographs were taken of thirty-seven patients at the close of each psychiatric interview in a mental health clinic to assist in a staff review. Besides aiding the staff in recognizing the clients, it was clear that the photographs contained the same type of information concerning problem areas that was noted by Coblentz (1964). Graham also reported that minimal posing occurred and that when it did occur, it was of diagnostic significance. He reports:

> Depression, anxiety, personality characteristics, and various other cues about behavior, manner and mood were clearly portrayed. The total appearance of the patient communicated a great deal of information and served as an invaluable aid in recall of content (from patient interviews).

Coblentz (1964) describes the use of photographs as diagnostic aids in a family mental health clinic. A policy of the clinic was to request a recent photograph of each of the family members coming to the clinic for treatment. The subsequent photographs provided much information regarding the more subtle nuances of the family interactions. He initially requested that families bring in family photographs to aid staff in remembering the families for later case review. He discovered that photographs had additional value as statements of clients' problem areas. In photos where father was out of the picture, it was likely that he was out of the picture in the family itself. Families that did not see themselves as units brought in individual photos. A narcissistic client gave the therapist a glamorous photo; a depressed client produced a sad photo; one death-phobic family produced a picture of themselves visiting a cemetery. A mother who was afraid that her fatherless son would grow up to be a juvenile delinquent or sexual deviant produced a photograph of him dressed as a choirboy.

Anderson and Malloy (1976) reported on a study using family photographs in treatment and training of clinicians at a family therapy clinic. They asked individual family members to bring in photos they thought were important statements about their family relationships. In discussing these photos, they used a warm-up technique in which the family members discussed their process of photo selection. In the actual viewing of these photos, the therapists paid attention to the order of presentation, the relative tempo of discussion, and the interest in and anxiety around each photograph. The therapists also considered the content and explored the images for spatial arrangement, closeness, formality, and presence or absence of members.

An interesting sidelight of this article is that when staff were asked to bring in photos as a way to identify and deal with negative practice issues in the clinic, there was much resistance. Members of the staff were fearful of being discovered as incompetent or mentally ill as a result of the photographic evidence. When these initial resistances were worked out and the photos brought in, they demonstrated that staff family relationships were similar to role relationships in the clinic. The awareness generated from these photos proved useful in drawing attention to and changing interpersonal staff behavior in the clinical setting.

Kulich and Goldberg (1978) investigated whether individuals at the opposite extremes of the introversion-extraversion scale would produce significantly different kinds of photographs when faced with the same subject matter (a male and female model). Judges rated the photographs produced by the extraverted subjects as significantly more "active" and "mobile."

Weiser (1975) states that "the crux of phototherapy (is): photography as a verb — learning about people's inner worlds, behavior and perceptions by skillfully observing *how* and *why* an individual chooses to select a certain photographic solution to meet his 'requirements'."

Krauss (1980c) has written about "the attributes of photographs that make them useful adjunctive tools for use by mental health professionals in the clinical setting." A number of therapeutic techniques are discussed relative to the special quality of photographs. He later (1981b) gave a number of examples that demonstrate the usefulness of photographs as both artifacts and metaphors. Mezibov (1981) reports on Krauss' writing about the use of photography in therapy to take client histories, as an aid to diagnosis, and as an adjunct to treatment.

Kaslow (1979) presents an example of successfully using "photo reconnaisance" to help uncover marital sex conflicts. She states that "photographs provide clues and highlight forerunners of current difficulties; they do not establish definitive causation." The question "who is in the bedroom with you?" often provides evidence of the symbolic power inherent in photographs to influence ("chaperone") couples. She states in conclusion: "Utilizing pictures provides a dynamic sense of the couple's history, physical contact and distance, sexual attractiveness or lack of same, and it is conducive to a growth and change orientation as it reflects pictorially the developments in and alterations achieved in the past."

In an early clinical application Muhl (1927) reported that the periodic study of patient snapshots over several years was helpful in bringing to light important clinical data regarding symptoms and conflicts for the patient.

Fox (1957) related an interesting case study using psychoanalysis to treat a young photographer. Fox stated that the patient had utilized his camera to gratify voyeuristic and exhibitionist impulses, as well as to achieve active visual focus on the external world. It is interesting to note the change of photographic subjects throughout the course of his analysis in relation to the verbal content of the analysis.

The literature on the diagnostic use of photographs as projective tests is very limited. Campbell and Burwen (1956) asked people to describe photos of fifty faces in terms of personality. They found consistent individual differences in responses. Cohen and Rau (1972), in a more successful study, asked women clients to pick one of forty-one facial expression photographs, which best described how they were feeling. They found that the task successfully separated normal from depressive women and did a better job of tapping the "momentary affective state" than interviews (where education and social class were not controlled). They suggest the use of this method especially when there are language and/or cultural barriers between the interviewer and the client.

Meer and Amon (1963) devised a test which used 100 facial photographs that were to be assessed by clients in terms of "liking the image" and "disliking the image." They concluded that the test showed patients more deviant than controls, that schizophrenics were more deviant than controls, that schizophrenics were more deviant than nonschizophrenics, and that patients with less deviancy (as measured by the test) were released relatively sooner. Females became less deviant as they improved, while males paradoxically did not become less deviant as they improved.

Gosciewski (1975), in his work with individual clients, reiterates some of the uses of photographs mentioned earlier in this introduction. He states that photographs provide information about the client's physical environment and offer good "there and then" or historical data to which counselors normally do not have access. Included in this information are data about the social involvement of the family at the neighborhood and community level as well. Photographs, furthermore, reveal or suggest client interaction patterns within these systems.

Photographs can be used with clients to build rapport, to make diagnoses, to verify or contradict client's perceptions, as projective devices, e.g. having clients caption photos, and as a means of more sharply delineating client self-perception through client selection and subsequent discussion of liked and disliked personal photos. Finally, photographs can serve as a transition in discussing "there and then" situations and "here and now" issues and concerns. He remarks:

> What we discovered in most instances was that not only did the photographs provide a wealth of incidental information about our clients, but also the clients came to feel more open in discussing the significant others and significant experience in their lives. . . . Early indications of the usefulness of photo counseling are promising and continued investigation is desirable. . . . As with so many other variations in counseling techniques, photo counseling affords a greater degree of interpersonal involvement in situations calling for heightened self-awareness and communication. (Gosciewski, 1975)

A FORM OF NONVERBAL COMMUNICATION BETWEEN CLIENT AND THERAPIST

Teller (1979) described photography as a visual medium with the unique characteristics of the visual mode of communication. Sontag (1977) reported that photographs furnish evidence and that the camera record incriminates or justifies. Sontag has stated that even though photographs may distort, there is an implicit assumption that the distortion is drawn from something that does or did exist.

Wolf (1976, 1978) has been most creative in his use of photography as nonverbal communication from client to therapist. His combination of psychoanalysis, drawing and photographs is used in unique therapy style, convenient to both brief and ongoing treatment modalities whose purpose is to allow unconscious material to rise to a conscious level at which it can be more easily recognized, dealt with, and resolved.

Ziller (1975) showed that unique psychological characteristics of a client can be demonstrated via photos. In a dramatic example (a photo taken by a client confined to a wheelchair), the viewer can readily see that even though the photo was taken in a group of people, no one in the group is acknowledging the presence of the wheelchair-confined photographer — a valid example of how "normal" people choose to ignore or turn their back on the physically handicapped. This is another example of the use of photos to help the counselor experience the world through the eyes of the client.

Combs and Ziller (1977), in counseling with college students, asked clients to take twelve photos that described themselves and to rank order them for discussion. They found that clients presented fewer pictures of themselves and more pictures of their family and their past than the control group. They concluded that clients more in a state of transition are more conflicted and have lower self-esteem. In review, this study suggests that client photos that lack images of themselves as active and in the present, demonstrate the limbo or "stuckness" of their perceived position.

Ziller and Smith (1977), using a phenomenological nonverbal approach to exploring perceptions of different student populations reported on three treatment conditions: (1) new students versus old students, (2) students permanently confined to wheelchairs versus normal students and (3) male versus female undergraduates. Results indicate that this approach is useful in freeing the individual from a total dependency on spoken language.

Ziller, Vera, and Camacho de Santoya (1981) reported work with children of poverty and affluence in Mexico City using photographs made in response to the question "who are you?" Content analysis revealed differences in the "psychological niche" of each group, with that of the affluent representing a "closed self-reinforcing system" while that of the poor (especially girls) representing a system of "survival within an extended group."

Krauss (1981a; 1982a; 1982b) has addressed himself to the theory of visual language in therapy and discusses photography as a means of "illuminating the metaphor." He discusses the nature of visual language and its metaphoric quality in the therapeutic relationship. He argues that the symbolic and imagistic nature of photographs (their nonlinearity) are less well defended against than language, and are accessed, processed and understood in different ways than verbal or written language. He also discusses predicate matching with visually dominant clients, and the use of visual language to teach clients new awareness and understanding.

DOCUMENTATION OF CHANGE

Akeret (1973) described photographs as "mirrors with memories" that can "pinpoint times of dramatic changes in looks, physical appearances, and feelings." Family albums also document changes in a family's life-style or orientation over the years; they are historical records of birth, marriages, death, etc. Reviewing these historical records is useful in helping the client to examine the various operations and relationships in the family and can help to correct distortions in an individual's life experience. In an article describing how "photographs and family albums can be used in marriage and family psychotherapy," Entin (1979) uses a systems approach to gather information about the family and its life cycle and to allow the family to understand what the photos portray about relationships in the family. He states that photographs are "links from the family's past to the present, and an affirmation of the traditions and ideals for the future."

In their work with families, Kaslow and Friedman (1977) have pointed out that even from a quantitative point of view, photos show important events and cycles in family life. For example, there are generally more photos of first-born children than of siblings and, during periods of stress, fewer photos are taken. They also suggest the use of older "there and then" (historical) photos of family to serve as a reminder that happier times have occurred in the family and, therefore, it may be possible to improve a presently painful family relationship. Their analysis indicates that consideration of size and placement of photos and pictures can yield significant data; e.g. if there are sexual problems in the marriage, are there religious or parental images in the bedroom? Furthermore, the act of discussing family photographs in the session acts to stimulate interactions among family members, expand awareness of others' roles and personalities, and can serve to sensitize the family to both their individual and collective appearance to the world. They conclude:

> Of value to the profession as a whole is that photo reconnaisance bridges the gap between two dominant schools of thought or opposing positions in psychotherapy on the role of historical data (the past) in the present and to the future. It utilizes pictures which recount the past as a stimulus and a focal point in the present to provide a sense of family history, and continuity and a foundation on which to help the family plan a meaningful, less conflicted, and more satisfying future. (Kaslow & Friedman, 1977).

In another use of family photographs, Ruben (1978) used photographs as documentation of perceived change by family members as result of therapy. She had each member create a family sculpture and photograph it at the beginning and end of treatment. She states the following:

> The picture is worth a thousand words. One can see in the nuclear family the coalitions

and separation or togetherness of the mother and father and the separation or togetherness of the siblings. It serves the same function as Minuchin's family map except that the therapist does not have to tease out the information to formulate the map because the family members have already done it in creating the family picture which allows the therapist to formulate hypotheses about which areas within the family function well and which may be dysfunctional. It also is a great help to the therapist in determining the therapeutic goals (Ruben, 1978).

Akeret (1973) describes his work with a young woman who was searching for a clue to her introversion and problem with obesity. In reviewing photographs of her past, the woman discovered a dramatic change in her appearance and apparent emotional condition in a photograph taken at about sixteen years of age. She later revealed to the therapist that at this age she began to change as a result of her boyfriend's pressuring her to have sexual intercourse with him. Progress in therapy occurred after the woman began addressing the problem through the help of the photo which documented the dramatic change in her.

Titus (1976) reported a study in which photographs were used to help couples in their transition to parenthood. Photographs were used to help document the change of the family image from one of a couple unit to one of a family unit.

Documenting change in therapy as a means of making clear that therapeutic change has occurred has been discussed by Zakem (1977). It is frequently encouraging or even a method of raising self-esteem in clients to go back and take a look at themselves beginning and concluding therapy.

PROLONGATION OF EXPERIENCES

Photographs are a record of our life experience; they trace our "roots" and as such, are frequently kept as keepsakes. We keep pictures of friends and relatives to be with us during absences and separations, and they recall loving memories of a friend or loved one who has died. Child welfare agencies and other social agencies who deal with foster children and children who are about to be adopted are beginning to prepare scrapbooks for these children of their foster parents, of their natural families, and of their new adoptive families. These are frequently children who are shifted from one placement to another; and these photographs help to ease the transition and are very often the only record of that child's life experiences up to that point.

Clients, especially those engaged in long-term therapy, frequently have a difficult time terminating therapy. The reasons are obvious. The close and intimate relationship with the therapist is often hard to terminate for both therapist and client, and it has been suggested that an exchange of photographs can enable both client and therapist to symbolically prolong the relationship.

Wikler (1977), as a supervisor of counselor training, has used photography as a way of dealing with the issues of separation between student-counselors and clients. The exchanging of photographs was useful in focusing on the issue of separation, helped to reduce the students' sense of loss and guilt, and let them experience the change with a sense of more continuity. Clients responded positively to this practice. Exchanged photographs can also serve to preserve memories in a concrete way. Wikler also noted that clients can bring in photos of deceased or otherwise unavailable family members or friends and use the photos as stimuli to explore termination issues in these relationships.

As part of the process of life review therapy with older people, Lewis and Butler (1974) used their photo albums. They found that the albums were useful in helping subjects to recall, integrate and sum up their lives. Most older individuals believe that photo reminiscence is a positive therapeutic experience. "Even persons with moderate brain damage can remember many details through pictures and keepsakes. On visits to older persons at home or in nursing homes or hospitals, the therapist can learn a good deal by commenting on pictures, mementos, or other personal items that are likely to have emotional meaning."

SELF-CONFRONTATION

A strong case for phototherapy is the use of photographs to provide a confrontation with one's self. The photograph is an excellent test of reality, and is a means that extends the "abilities of the eye and brain to see, evaluate, and judge the external world as selected by the client's self" (Zakem, 1977). Photographs can be used to show a person what he or she looks like, as in an alcoholic or drunken state, or what he or she could look like, as in a groomed or improved state. Many of the studies using photography as a self-confrontation approach have operated using the theory that if individuals can see themselves as objectively as others see them, then they will use this new information to help themselves change for the better. There have been positive results using this approach.

Greenleigh (1974) advocates the use of media to aid in visual self-confrontation with middle-aged clients to help them recognize their individual and unique value. Among other media, videotape and family albums are recommended in this process.

Trusso (1979) reported on the use of instant self-photography as part of a holistic therapy practice. He states that this process "offers several unique opportunities ranging from greater depth understanding of personal body configurations, to immediate feedback unencumbered by either verbal codification or therapist specific prejudices."

Spire (1973) used "photographic-self image confrontation" (PSIC) with twelve female chronic schizophrenics over a six-week period in an institutional setting. Each person was photographed and interviewed. The interview included such questions as: "Who is the person in the picture? What do you like about the picture? What do you dislike? What would you like to change? Does this picture remind you of anyone else?" This method of treatment was seen as very successful in inducing patients to explore their self-concepts with their therapists. Spire concludes as follows:

> To determine if PSIC could produce positive behavioral changes in chronically ill schizophrenic female patients, I administered the Adjective Check List and the Draw-A-Person Test to study the patients prior to their participation in the PSIC sessions and again after the sessions had been completed. In addition, ward staff attendants rated patients on the Hospital Adjustment Scale in a like fashion. . . . We found that 75 percent of the patients who participated in PSIC improved in the area of communications and interpersonal relations. This was statistically significant at the .01 level of confidence. Approximately 60 percent of the patients improved in the area relating to care of self and social responsibility; this was significant at the .05 level of confidence. In the area of work, recreation, and activities, two-thirds of the patients showed improvement which was significant at the .01 level of confidence. . . . Over 90% of the patients showed a positive behavioral change as they demonstrated a keener awareness of body boundaries, regarded themselves in a more positive manner, and relinquished some of their negative self-aspects. This change was significant at the .01 level of confidence (as evaluated from the Draw-A-Person Test).

Hall (1980) used his skills as a photographer and therapist to help improve subjects' self-images and self-esteem. He photographed eight women with the intent of evaluating the results of this process. Each subject was photographed and given a number of activities to assess their feelings around their personal appearance, how they described themselves as physical beings, and who were identified as significant others in their world. Subjects were then photographed again approximately ten days later. "Having patients view photographs of themselves has been identified by those who use photo therapy as 'self-confrontation.' In this study, the photographs which were given to the subjects were produced with the goal of being pleasing to them. This technique may be thought of as 'controlled self-confrontation.' Potential clinical uses are altering self-perceptions, improving self-esteem, enhancing involvement in treatment, exploring roles, and observing interaction processes."

Cornelison and Arsenian (1960) studied responses of a small sample of patients in a psychiatric setting when they were photographed with Polaroid cameras and immediately interviewed with regard to the photographs. Patients who changed as a result of the photo self-confrontation experience (most patients) showed expanded self-concept or at least a limited self-appreciation. The authors concluded that this method can be successfully used as an adjunct to therapy, and that it seems to bring some psychotics into better contact with reality. The authors conclude:

> Draw-A-Person Tests were obtained in pre- and post-test sessions and also midway in the series. In all but one case, these drawings showed progressively more realistic representation of the human body. The final drawings suggest that the patients' feelings of animalness, inanimateness, or dissolution had diminished and that their sense of the body's integrity and basic humaness had increased. . . . Photographic self-image experi-

ence may afford an adjunct to psychotherapy with seriously disturbed persons.

Fryrear and his colleagues (see Chapter 5) have carried out several studies on photographic self-confrontation with varying success. The studies all have in common the viewing of self-portraits by clients in an attempt to provide the clients with more visual information about themselves than they may have already. The studies have shown more success with children and adolescent boys than with adolescent girls.

PHOTOTHERAPY TRAINING

Krauss (1979b) created a training model that covered the areas of "self-concept, individual photographs, family photographs, photographs used as projective devices, photo essays and the uses of photographs in termination, separation and grief work." In the course announcement (1978) he stated, "The purpose is to show how photography can be used to aid self-discovery to expand personal and interpersonal awareness, and as a tool for working with clients in other than strictly verbal modes."

A summary of the research from the development of the phototherapy training model was reported by Krauss in 1980(b). As a result of training, a treatment group was found to exhibit significant differences from a matched control group in their ability to make more useful comments and observations about a number of photographs. An interesting note about this study was that "No significant correlation between sex, age, interest in photography, or work experience was found for either the treatment group or the control group for individual item responses."

PREVIEW OF REMAINING CHAPTERS

In this chapter we have reviewed some of the many reported uses of photography in mental health and related areas. We certainly have not mentioned all the published accounts. We have sought to give the reader both a sense of phototherapy literature history and its varied domain. In the chapters to follow, the authors will provide more detailed information related to their particular interests. Having read this introductory chapter, you will recognize the names of the contributors. We have summarized the work of some, and alluded to others. All of the contributors have written original chapters for this volume, and the chapters represent the "state of the art" of phototherapy at present.

Chapter 2, by Douglas Stewart, is a history of photography as it relates to phototherapy. Within the historical context of photography, Stewart attempts to give the reader a sense of the personal nature of photography and to show why photography is a particularly appropriate tool for therapy.

David Krauss, in Chapter 3, discusses the relationships among reality, photography and psychotherapy. This theoretical discussion will prove to be a sound basis for an understanding of visual modes of therapy.

In Chapter 4, Krauss narrows his discussion to the underlying assumptions of phototherapy and its visual symbolism. He provides a short review of the use of visuals in contacting and comprehending the world, and in creating symbols. He presents some therapeutic applications as he seeks to "illuminate the visual metaphor."

Chapter 5 is concerned with another aspect of therapy, self-confrontation. Jerry L. Fryrear reviews photography as self-confrontation and attempts to arrive at a satisfactory explanation as to the value of visual self-confrontation.

Robert C. Ziller and his colleagues have developed a method of phototherapy, which they describe in Chapter 6. Their clients use photography to describe to themselves and to the therapist how they perceive their "psychological niche" in the environment. They report on a series of studies using the method.

Chapter 7 is devoted to the use of photographs in family therapy. Alan D. Entin discusses family photographs as links to the past, and relates family phototherapy to the family systems theory of Bowen.

Chapter 8, by Joel Walker, illustrates the use of photographs as a catalyst in individual psychotherapy and gives case illustrations of the role of photographs in the therapeutic processes of rapport, affect, resistance, transference, and working through conflicts.

An art therapist and psychoanalyst, Robert Wolf, describes instant phototherapy with children and adolescents in Chapter 9. He reviews the technique of instant phototherapy, points out the implications for treatment of acting-out disorders and learning disabled youngsters, and describes the nature of the treatment process.

Judy Weiser, who has worked with native, handicapped, and otherwise "different" people, describes her phototherapy in Chapter 10. She relates phototherapy to anthropological concepts and illustrates her work with a case report of a deaf youngster of native American ancestry.

Chapter 11, by Brian Zakem, relates phototherapy to the broader field of psychotherapy. Zakem provides an integration of mental health service components, the basic components of phototherapy, and the options the contemporary phototherapist has among the various visual techniques.

David Krauss addresses us again in Chapter 12, this time with coauthor Ansel Woldt, reporting on a training program that they have developed for phototherapists. They offer practical advice on equipment needs, class outlines, and behavioral objectives.

The book concludes with a brief summary by the editors, with a discussion of major points covered by the contributors and apparent trends in the practice of phototherapy.

REFERENCES

Akeret, R.V. *Photoanalysis.* New York: Peter H. Wyden, Inc., 1973.

Ammerman, M.S. and Fryrear, J.L. Photographic enhancement of children's self esteem. *Psychology in the Schools,* 1975, *12* (3), 319-325.

Anderson, C.M. and Malloy, E.S. Family photographs: In treatment and training. *Family Process,* 1976, *15* (2), 259-264.

Aronson, D.W., and Graziano, A.M. Improving elderly clients' attitudes through photography. *The Gerontologist,* 1976, *16* (4), 363-476. ·

Campbell, D.T., and Burwen, L.S. Trait judgments from photographs as a projective device. *Journal of Clinical Psychology,* 1956, *12,* 215-221.

Coblentz, A.L. Use of photographs in a family mental health clinic. *American Journal of Psychiatry,* 1964, *121,* 601-611.

Cohen, B.D., and Rau, J.H. Nonverbal technique for measuring affect using facial expression photographs as stimuli. *Journal of Consulting and Clinical Psychology,* 1972, *38*(3), 449-452.

Combs, J.H., and Ziller, R.C. Photographic self-concept of counselees. *Journal of Counseling Psychology,* 1977, *24*(5), 452-455.

Cornelison, F.S., and Arsenian, J. A study of the response of psychotic patients to photographic self-image experience. *Psychiatric Quarterly,* 1960, *34*(1), 1-8.

Entin, A.D. Reflection of families. *Photo Therapy Quarterly,* 1979, *2*(2), 19-21.

Fox, H.M. Body image of a photographer. *Journal of the American Psychoanalytic Association,* 1957, *5,* 93-107.

Fryrear, J.L. A selective, nonevaluative review of research on photo therapy. *Photo Therapy Quarterly,* 1980, *2*(3), 7-9.

Fryrear, J.L., Nuell, L.R., and Ridley, S.D. Photographic self-concept enhancement of male juvenile delinquents. *Journal of Consulting and Clinical Psychology,* 1974, *42*(6), 915.

Fryrear, J.L., Nuell, L.R., and White, P. Enhancement of male juvenile delinquents' self concepts through photographed social interactions. *Journal of Clinical Psychology,* 1977, *33*(3), 833-838.

Fryrear, J.L., and Fleshman, R. (Eds.). *Videotherapy in mental health.* Springfield, IL: Charles C Thomas, Publisher, 1981.

Gilman, S. (Ed.). *The face of madness.* New York: Brunner/Mazel, 1976.

Gilman, S. *Seeing the insane.* New York: John Wiley and Sons in association with Brunner/Mazel, 1982.

Gosciewski, W.F. Photo counseling. *Personnel and Guidance Journal,* 1975, *53*(8), 600-604.

Graham, J.R. The use of photographs in psychiatry. *Canadian Psychiatric Association Journal,* 1967, 12, 425.

Greenleigh, L. Facing the challenge of change in middle age. *Geriatrics,* 1974, 29(11), 61-68.

Hall, D.G. Photography as a learning experience in self-perception. Doctoral dissertation, University of Michigan, 1980.

Hattersley, R. *Discover yourself through photography.* New York: Morgan and Morgan, 1971.

Hattersley, R. 30 Ways photography is good for you. *Popular Photography,* February, 1980, 87-127.

Hedges, R.E. Photography and self-concept. *Audiovisual Instruction.* 1972, 17(5), 26-28.

Jaffe, D.J., and Bressler, D.E. The use of guided imagery as an adjunct to medical diagnosis and treatment. *Journal of Humanistic Psychology,* 1980, *20*(4), 47-59.

Kaslow, F. What personal photos reveal about marital sex conflicts. *Journal of Marital and Sex Therapy,* 1979, *5*(2), 134-141.

Kaslow, F. and Friedman, J. Utilization of family photos and movies in family therapy. *Journal of Marriage and Family Counseling,* 1977, *3*(1), 19-25.

Krauss, D. A summary of characteristics of photographs which make them useful in counseling and therapy. *Camera Lucida,* 1980, *1*(2), 2-12.(c)

Krauss, D. Photo therapy course offered at Kent State (edited by B. Zakem). *Photo Therapy Quarterly,* 1979, *2*(1), 12-13.(a)

Krauss, D. Photography, imaging, and visually referent language in therapy: Illuminating the metaphor. *Camera Lucida,* 1982. *1*(c5), 58-63 (a).

Krauss, D. Insight and Outlook: Symbol and Metaphor in Phototherapy. Paper presented at the American Psychological Association National Convention, 1982 (b).

Krauss, D. On Photography: Its uses in psychotherapy. Paper presented at the American Psychological Association National Convention, 1981 (b).

Krauss, D. Phototherapy overview. Unpublished lecture given at Kent State University phototherapy training workshop, 1980 (a).

Krauss, D. The uses of still photography in counseling and therapy: Development of a training model. Doctoral dissertation, Kent State University, 1979 (b).

Krauss, D. The uses of still photography in counseling and therapy: Development of a training model (illustrated dissertation abstract). *Photo Therapy Quarterly,* 1980, *2*(3), 12-13 (b).

Krauss, D. Utilizing photographs and visual language in therapy: Illuminating the metaphor. *Photo Therapy,* 1981, *2*(4), 6-7 (a).

Kulich, R.J., and Goldberg, R.W. Differences in the production of photographs: A potential assessment technique. *Perceptual and Motor Skills,* 1978, 47, 223-229.

Levinson, R. Psychodynamically oriented photo therapy. *Photo Therapy Quarterly,* 1979, *2*(2), 14-16.

Lewis, M.E., and Butler, R.N. Life review therapy. *Geriatrics Quarterly,* Nov., 1974, 165-173.

Loellbach, M. Case illustration. *Photo Therapy Quarterly,* 1978, *1*(3), 2-3.

McDougall-Treacy, G. The person as camera experience. *Photo Therapy Quarterly,* 1979, *2*(2), 16-18.

McKinney, J.P. Photo counseling. *Children Today,* 1979, *8*(1), 29.

Meer, B., and Amon, A.H. Photo preference test (PPT) as a measure of mental status for hospitalized psychiatric patients. *Journal of Consulting Psychology,* 1963, *27*(4), 283-293.

Mezabov, D. Photographs as therapy. American Psychological Association Monthly Science Summary #192, November, 1981 (Summary of D. Krauss' "On photography: Uses in psychotherapy" presented at 1981 national convention of American Psychological Association).

Milford S., Swank, P., and Fryrear, J.L. Enhancement of self esteem, social skills and grooming in institutionalized adolescent boys through photography. Unpublished paper, 1981.

Milgram, S. The image freezing machine. *Psychology Today,* January, 1977, *108*, 5-54.

Miller, M.F. Responses of psychiatric patients to their photographed images. *Diseases of the Nervous System,* 1962, *23*, 296-298.

Muhl, A.M. Notes on the use of photography in checking up on unconscious conflicts. *Psychoanalytic Review,* 1927, *14*, 329-331.

Myers, E.S. Photographic images as a visual induction into an alpha and/or altered state of consciousness. Doctoral dissertation, Boston University, 1977.

Nelson-Gee, E. Learning to be: A look into the use of therapy with Polaroid photography as a means of recreating the development of perception and the ego. *Art Psychotherapy,* 1975, *2*(2), 159-174.

Nicoletti, D.J. An investigation into the effects of a self-directed photography experience upon the self-concept of fourth grade students. Doctoral dissertation, Syracuse University, 1972.

Poli, K. Photoprobes. *Popular Photography,* 1979, *85*(3), 91; 134.

Ruben, A.G. The family picture. *Journal of Marriage and Family Counseling,* 1978, *4*(3), 25-28.

Smith, J.R. Taking portrait photographs of children in therapy. *Photo Therapy Quarterly,* 1978, *1*(4), 1-2.

Sontag, S. *On photography.* New York: Farrar, Strauss and Giroux, 1977.

Spire, R.H. Photographic self image confrontation. *American Journal of Nursing,* 1973, *73*(7), 1207-1210.

Stewart, D. Photography and psychology join hands. Unpublished paper, Northern Illinois University, 1978.

Teller, A. Some questions for photo therapy. *Photo Therapy Quarterly,* 1979, *2*(2), 12-13.

Teller, A., Langsan, N., and Levinson, R. Photography in the classroom: A workbook. Springfield IL: Illinois Arts Council, 1975.

Titus, S.L. Family photographs and the transition to parenthood. *Journal of Marriage and the Family,* 1976, *38*(3), 525-530.

Trusso, J. Some uses of instant photography in holistic therapy. *Photo Therapy Quarterly,* 1979, *2* (1), 14-15.

Turner-Hogan, P. The use of group photo therapy in the classroom. *Photo Therapy,* 1981, *2*(4), 13.

Tyding, K. Instamatic therapy. *Human Behavior,* 1973, February.

Vardell, M., McClellan, L. and Fryrear, J.L. A structured group phototherapy program and its use with adjudicated adolescent girls. *Phototherapy,* 1982, *3*(2), 8-11.

Vogel, R.K. The effects of an audiovisual relaxation training program upon pulse rate, skin temperature and anxiety. Doctoral dissertation, Boston College, 1977.

Walker, J. See and tell. *Photo Therapy Quarterly,* 1980, *2*(3), 14-15.

Walker, J. 1981 update: The photograph as a catalyst in psychotherapy. Unpublished paper, Toronto, 1981.

Weal, E. Photo psychology. *Innovations,* 1980, *6*(3), 13-15.

Weiser, J. Phototherapy: photography as a verb. *The B.C. Photographer,* Fall, 1975, 33-36.

White, M. Extended perception through photography and suggestion. In H. Otto and J. Mann (Eds.), *Ways of growth.* New York: Viking Press, 1969.

White, M. Varieties of responses to photographs. *Aperture,* 1962, *10*(3), 116-128.

Wikler, M.E. Using photographs in the termination phase. *Social Work,* 1977, *22*(4), 318-319.

Williams, R.D., and Williams, R.C.M. Photography as a bridge between institution and community: a preventive intervention. *Photo Therapy,* 1981, *2*(4), 8-12.

Wolf, R. The polaroid technique: Spontaneous dialogues from the unconscious. *Art Psychotherapy,* 1976, *3*(3/4), 197-201.

Zakem, B. Photo therapy: A developing psychotherapeutic approach. Unpublished paper, Ravenswood Community Mental Health Center, Chicago, 1977.

Ziller, R. Psychology and photography. *The B.C. Photographer,* Fall, 1975, 7.

Ziller, R., Vera, H., and Camacho de Santoya, C. Understanding children of poverty or affluence through auto-photographic metaphor. Paper presented at the national convention of the American Psychological Association, 1981.

Ziller, R. and Smith, R.A. A phenomenological utilization of photographs. *Journal of Phenomenological Psychology,* 1977, *7,*(2), 172-182.

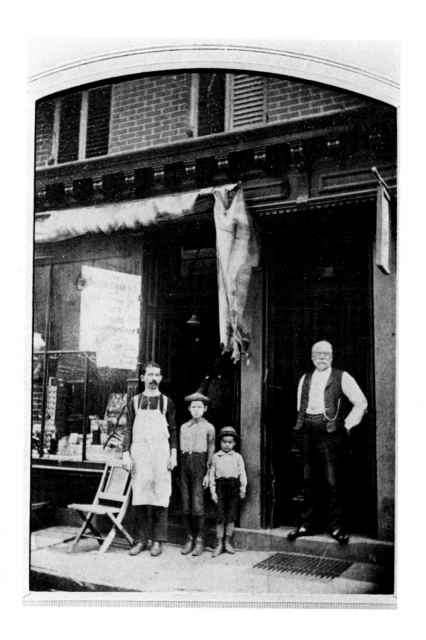

Collection of David A. Krauss

Chapter 2

Phototherapy: Looking into the History of Photography

DOUGLAS STEWART

INTRODUCTION

ALTHOUGH the contemporary practice of phototherapeutic techniques does not require skills in the craft of photography per se, most mental health professionals do have at least some passing acquaintance with the phenomena of making and looking at photographs. Indeed the general public has been interested and enthusiastic about photography since its inception. Over time the process of picture-making has become increasingly simple for amateur photographers due to the increasingly sophisticated technology of this century, allowing us in this day and age to look through a viewfinder, press a button and have a finished print in ninety seconds. Obviously, in the beginnings of photography the process was much slower and more arduous. Additionally, while many mental health professionals may use photography as part of their intervention strategies, only a few may have a more general background of the history and development of this medium as a force in our culture. The purpose of this chapter is to give the reader a general historical understanding of this seemingly technical and yet personal form of expression and communication, and to show why photography can be a particularly well-suited vehicle to aid in assessment, diagnosis, and treatment in the therapeutic process. It attempts to give the reader a more complete picture of the interface of these two disciplines, which at first glance appear to be so different.

ADVENT OF A NEW MEDIUM

The years 1839 and 1856 were auspicious ones in the history and development of phototherapy. In France, 1839 saw the inception of photography with the first public announcement of Daguerre's "daguerreotype."

The author wishes to thank David Krauss for his aid and encouragement in the compilation of this chapter.

25

In England, that same year, Fox-Talbot annouced his "Calotype," the forerunner of the modern negative-positive photographic process, while noted scientist Herschel named these new pictorial methods "photography" (Craven, 1975). According to Gernsheim (1965),

> Probably no other invention ever captured the imagination of the public to such an extent and conquered the world with such lightening rapidity as the daguerreotype. (p. 59).

Seventeen years later, in 1856, Freud was born in Moravia (now part of Czechoslovakia), and the English psychiatrist and amateur photographer Diamond presented his illustrated paper on his theories of the uses of photography in psychiatry to the London Royal Society of Medicine (Gilman, 1976). It remained for the twentieth century, however, to synthesize these distinctive events into a new discipline called phototherapy.

With photography now being over 140 years old, it is hard to imagine the excitement with which its invention was greeted in 1839. Coinciding with the rapid growth of the middle class in the industrialized nations, the camera promised to the many what only the privileged few had previously been able to afford from the artist's brush: a visual likeness of themselves. Within a few years of their introduction, photographs were being made and purchased on a vast scale; for example, Gernsheim (1965) reported that in 1853 an estimated three million daguerreotypes were made in the United States alone. For the first time it was possible for the common man to have a personal history in visual form.

As the new medium developed technically from the daguerreotype and calotype to the tintype (photographs on blackened tin), the photographic portrait became increasingly popular. More and more portrait studios opened — New York alone had nearly 100 in the early 1850s (Gernsheim, 1965) — and prices became lower. In the last years of the daguerreotype in the late 1850s, operators were making multiple images with multi-lensed cameras, reducing prices for the delicate silver-and-copper images to a low of 12 1/2 cents each. The subsequent invention of the even more popular tintype offered sturdiness, even lower prices, and portability: the era of the "snapshot" was not far off.

Although still requiring elaborate multi-lensed cameras and processing equipment, the invention of the paper *cartes de visite* (visiting cards) by the Frenchman Disderi in 1854 (Gernsheim, 1965) lowered costs even further and thereby increased the already considerable infusion of personal images throughout the culture. For example, in about 1855, he was turning out nearly 2400 photographs a day from his Paris studio. It must be of interest to the phototherapist that the albums in which the *cartes de visite* of friends and family were kept were the forerunner of the contemporary family album.

The public soon discovered, however, that having one's likeness in permanent form was a mixed advantage. According to Gernsheim (1965):

> The realization that the camera revealed the sitter with uncompromising truth, dispelling cherished illusions of youth and beauty, was disconcerting at first, particularly to women. The demands of the sitter for a good likeness and at the same time a beautiful

portrait were — and still are — seldom compatible. (p. 64).

Freud himself conceded in a letter to Jung in 1907 that "In the last fifteen years I have never willingly sat for a photographer because I am too vain to countenance my physical deterioration" (Freud-House catalog, 1975, p. 38).

Photography did not simply limit itself to a role of portraitist for Everyman, but soon established itself as an integral component in the development of modern western culture. Lyons (1966) credits the critic Dadakidir Hartman with pointing out in 1910 that the results of photography permeate all intellectual phases of our life. Hartman contended that through the illustration of newspapers, books, magazines, business circulars, and advertisements, objects that previous to Daguerre's invention were not represented pictorally had become "common property" (p. 13). As early as 1910, therefore, the cultural impact of the photograph had already become sufficiently pervasive as to be almost invisible.

This influence, however, was not necessarily accompanied by clarity of purpose or function. Indeed, as Craven (1975) states in his preface to *Object and Image*.

> Photography is by all odds our most common picture making process. When its effect on the way we see things is considered, it is also quite likely our least understood one. (p. vii)

As an entirely new way of producing images and symbols, photography did not lend itself to ready analysis with the traditional critical tools so useful with other pictorial media. There were present in the new medium levels and dimensions of pictorial illusions that were sufficiently unlike prior graphic imagery as to require new critical approaches and understandings.

One of the most prevalent and persistent of those illusions was the collapsed aesthetic distance between object and image, when compared with painting, drawing, etching, or other graphic media. As Friedlander observes in the foreword to *Storyville Portraits* (1970), "Well, the one thing about the camera is that in a hundredth of a second or less it renders everything . . . it really is a sort of magic" (p. 12).

Editor Szarkowski goes on to theorize that:

> Perhaps much of the magic — the mystery — lies in this: a good photograph convinces us that it does indeed render everything; we would not know how to add to its completeness. And yet half a dozen photographs made in a given room at a given hour will each describe a different reality. . . . Photography has enabled us to explore the richness of that swarming, shifting, four-dimensional continuum that we choose to call reality. It has shown us that what is "out there" is not a catalog of discreet facts and Ptolmaic measurements, but a sea of changing relationships. (p. 12)

This realistic aspect of the photographic image, however, has left us with a peculiar set of problems as Craven (1975) explains:

> People readily believe that the photographic image is indeed a re-creation of the original object, and photographers, on the whole seem content to let this naive assumption go unchallenged. A photograph signifies the "real," thus it becomes a symbol of truth. The fact that a photograph presents only an *illusion* of reality may often go unnoticed. (pp. 10-11)

It is not a long conceptual leap from accepting the photography as reality to believing that photographing subject matter is tantamount to possessing it as one's own, or that objects and people photographed somehow become extensions of one's own domain. Sontag (1977) addresses this issue when she contends that, "To collect photographs is to collect the world," adding that, "To photograph is to appropriate the thing photographed. It means putting oneself into a certain relation to the world that feels like knowledge — and, therefore, like power" (p. 3).

The late Diane Arbus, a photographer speaking of her own work (1972), emphasizes this point when she reports:

> There's a kind of power thing about the camera. I mean everyone knows you've got some edge. You're carrying some slight magic which does something to them. It fixes them in a way. (p. 13)

Nor is Arbus alone in ascribing possessive abilities to Holmes' (1859) "mirror with a memory." As quoted by Hall (1968), Minor White, author, critic, teacher, editor, and photographer, describes his camera work thusly:

> To take photographs. Such was the entry point into photography. Along the creek beds and waterfalls *seeing* was always possession and *camera* affirmed ownership. Since then other modes, other doors have superseded. . . . The greed, however, has never really disappeared. Ownership seems to be the force that opens all the other doors. (p. 16)

If connection and possession are two of the motivators for photographing, then one might assume that control of the subject is also a motivating factor. Sontag (1977) agrees, stating that a photograph "is part of, an extension of that subject; and a potent means of acquiring it, of gaining control over it" (p. 155). She argued that photography is acquisition in the form of surrogate possession of a prized person or thing; and also that it is a consumer's relationship to events in which we have artifacts of an event, even though we were not a participant in it. She also pointed out that through image-making and duplicating machines we acquire information *about* things, rather than the experience *of* them.

It could be theorized from the above that photography can function both as a facilitator of heightened informational awareness and as a catalyst of alienation; that is, by functioning as a McLuhanesque "extension of man," photography is increasingly able to expose us to a wider range of once-removed visual experiences than ever before. At the same time, however, because of photography's realistic illusionary quality, we are apt to settle for the illusion rather than the reality, leaving us further isolated from first-hand experience. As McLuhan (1964) points out, "Thus the world itself becomes a sort of museum of objects that have been encountered before in some other medium" (p. 198).

Endowed with this kind of power to mold and change, the act of photographing can become its own reason for being, its own rationale. Sontag

(1977) agrees that:

> A photograph is not just the result of an encounter between an event and a photographer; picture-taking is an event in itself, and one with ever more preemptory rights — to interfere with, to invade, or to ignore whatever is going on . . . while real people are out there killing themselves or other real people, the photographer stays behind his or her camera, creating a tiny element of another world; the image-world that bids to outlast us all. (p. 11)

To which Arbus (1972) adds from her own experience:

> I have this funny thing which is that I'm never afraid when I'm looking in the ground glass (of the camera). This person could be approaching with a gun or something like that and I'd have my eyes glued to the finder and it wasn't like I was really vulnerable. It just seemed terrific what was happening. I mean I'm sure there are limits. God knows, when the troops start advancing on me, you do approach that stricken feeling where you perfectly well can get killed. (pp. 12-13)

Given photography's apparent powers of illusion, control, and possession — all activities of the mind — it seems that the ingredients were present for an expanding relationship with psychotherapy.

EARLY USE OF PHOTOGRAPHY IN THERAPY

The earliest documented use of photography in psychotherapy, was, as noted earlier, by Diamond, an English psychiatrist and amateur photographer (Gilman, 1976). A physiognomist and resident superintendent of the Female Department of the Surrey County Lunatic Asylum, Diamond photographed his patients as a clinical aid in identifying various diagnosed types of mental illness. According to Gilman (1976), Diamond suggests these three benefits of photography relative to the treatment of mental illness:

> It can record the appearance of the mentally ill for study (ascribing to the theories of the physiognomy of insanity presented at that period); it can be used in the treatment of the mentally ill through the presentation of an accurate self-image; and it can record the visages of patients to facilitate identification for later admission and treatment. (pp. 7-8)

Diamond discovered that by photographing patients during stages of their treatment, he was able to show change in their appearance. Of primary interest to contemporary phototherapists, he also discovered that these photographic records of changes in appearance had both a positive therapeutic value when shown to the patients and were an instructive function for the staff. Diamond presented an illustrated paper on his work to London's Royal Society of Medicine in 1856. Despite his contentions that photography was useful in therapy, when Diamond opened his own private asylum in 1858 at Twickenham House, Middlesex, he apparently no longer photographed his patients.

In the 1870s, also according to Gilman (1976), the inmates of the orphanages administered by a Dr. Barnardo were photographed "to record their altered physical development in their new environment" (p. 10). In the 1880s,

Hood photographed inmates at Bethlehem Asylum (Gilman, 1976) a practice that by then was apparently not uncommon:

> In fact, the taking of portraits has become one of the pleasures of which the patients cheerfully partake in our lunatic asylums; and helps, in combination with the various other alleviations studied by humane superintendents to diversify and cheer the days passed in necessary seclusion from the busier, but scarcely happier world, without. One incidental effect of these artistical amusements is to draw the attention of the patients themselves to their own costume and figure; and this direction of their notice may lead to salutary results. (p. 10)

Despite these promising beginnings, a documented, systematic body of knowledge and literature with regard to the use of photography in therapeutic settings is just now being developed.

THE SNAPSHOT

Many of the images that clients bring to the therapeutic setting can be considered "snapshots;" and perhaps no form of photography is so widely practiced, yet is so little understood. Most of the approximately four *billion* photographs turned out yearly by an estimated 60 million amateurs' cameras in the United States alone (Sturr, 1979) can probably be labeled "snapshots."

According to Kouwenhoven (1974), the term originated around 1808 in English hunting jargon referring to a hurried shot, taken without deliberate aim. Herschel, who had labeled the new medium "photography" in 1839 (Craven, 1975), was also apparently the first to use the term "snapshot" in 1860 in relation to photography (Kouwenhoven, 1974).

Despite this historical precedent, however, the term continues to mean different things to different people. *Webster's Seventh New Collegiate Dictionary* (1963) defines "snapshot" as "A casual photograph made by rapid exposure, usually with a small hand-held camera" (p. 825). Critic and teacher Jonathan Green (1974) states that "the word 'snapshot' is the most ambiguous, controversial word in photography since the word 'art' " (p. 3). Photographer Wendy Snyder MacNeil (1974) believes that "Snapshots, photographs from family albums, are today's cave paintings, born of the same urges, rituals" (p. 58).

Another concept of the snapshot is that of historian Michael Lesy (1976), author of *Wisconsin Death Trip,* who states in his article in *Afterimage*:

> I think that snapshots are the private thoughts about love and family life which this culture has chosen to express semi-publicly. They are like the conversations that passed between the men in Paul Bunyan's logging camp during a winter that was so cold that the words froze to the walls and rafters.
>
> I think snapshots are primarily psychological documents. They may be understood aesthetically, anthropologically, and historically as well. But I think that because they are personally and privately made images whose information is graphic, tacit, factual, and allusive, they must first be deciphered as if they were dreams, before they can be understood as if they were primitive paintings, poems, or excerpts from letters.

Photographer Lisette Model (1974), who has photographed people for most of her professional career, states that:

> I am a passionate lover of the snapshot, because of all photographic images it comes closest to truth. The snapshot is a specific spiritual moment. It cannot be willed or desired to be achieved. It simply happens, to certain people and not to others. (p. 6)

Peter Bunnell (1972), writer/critic/historian, has addressed the apparently disparate relationship between the ease with which snapshots are produced and the level of their emotional significance. According to Bunnell:

> Perhaps the most fascinating of all the aspects of portraiture is that which concerns the rapport between the subject photographed and the photographer. In this context a consideration of the snapshot is illuminating. From a position of sophistication these pictures are viewed as a kind of primitivism, not unlike children's drawings. But this is only one aspect which should interest us. For while the facile way in which such pictures are made eludes considered thought, the majority of them represent a pictorial record of the most private of human relations between people. It is a curious fact, but it seems that serious photographers make very few conventional snapshots.
>
> Because snapshot photographs represent pure picture making, where the configuration of things matters little and the content is obvious and unrestricted, their meaning is considered minimal by those not actually involved in the process. But for the individual who wished to take the picture, or for the person who wished to retain it, there is no more intimate and ultimately successful portrait in existence. The adequacy of meaning in the snapshot rests singularly on the psychology of privacy and the intensity of human reasoning. (unpaged)

From the variety of thoughts about the snapshot by those professionally involved with the medium of photography, it can be seen that the snapshot has acquired both critical attention and a respected place within the medium. It has also played a significant role in the sociological development of our culture, a role that remained largely unarticulated until the latter third of this century, when the social ramifications of the snapshot became more apparent.

It should be noted that the snapshot became possible through the development of small, inexpensive, and simple hand-held cameras, exemplified by the first Kodak®, introduced by the George Eastman Company in 1888. With this apparatus, the user took 100 pictures and returned the camera and $10.00 to the company for processing and reloading (Newhall, 1949). The following year, Eastman introduced flexible roll film (Gernsheim, 1969) and the era of snapshot photography was launched. Eastman advertised, "You press the button, we do the rest" (Newhall, 1949), and millions of new photographers around the world *did*. (See Figure 2-1).

A variety of approaches were taken by the users of these new visual appendages once they were free from the cumbersome tripods and glass plates of an earlier era. The formal visit to the portrait studio in the Victorian era became the do-it-yourself lark on the beach in the Snapshot era. The act of photographing was taken from the few and given to the many — photography had gone public. As Shortenwyde (1943) pointed out, "For the first time, the act of photograph*ing* may have became as important as the resultant image" (p. 173).

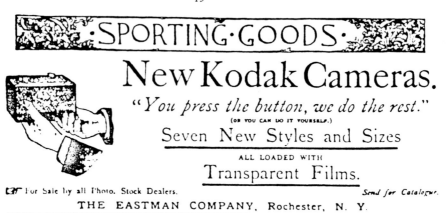

Figure 2-1. Kodak advertisement of the late 1800s.

The societal fallout from this post-1888 deluge of personal images has been enormous. It seems more than coincidence that the Victorian era ended with the birth of the snapshot. Halpren (1974) comments on this point:

> The recalcitrant hand camera spontaneously and accidentally generated its own informal style. This radically photographic style hinted at visual and cultural truths that were far removed from the stereotypes which gave form to the Victorian portrait. The snapshot began to characterize the family in terms of interaction. No longer did father stand behind and above his family as the ruling patriarch. The snapshot allowed each member of the family to acquire an identity defined by his relationship with others and his physical surroundings. The snapshot could still record the posed moment, but it could also capture the fleeting expression and candidly look at the ongoing life of the nuclear family as it was actually experienced.
>
> The family albums of my great-grandparents are filled with serious and severe people looking as if they were bringing in their souls to judgment. The snapshots in the albums of my parents show Mom and Dad throwing snowballs at each other in the storm of 1947. (pp. 66-67)

In order to better understand the cultural milieu that the snapshot helped to create, and from which phototherapy has subsequently emerged, it may be helpful to refer to Kouwenhoven's (1974) explanation of the impact of the snapshot upon our collective vision:

> Unwittingly, amateur snapshooters were revolutionizing mankind's way of seeing. We do not yet realize, I think, how fundamentally snapshots altered the way people saw one another and the world around them by reshaping our conceptions of what is real and therefore of what is important. We tend to see only what the pictorial conventions of our time are calculated to show us. (p. 107)
>
> Before photography, reality was history, and history was very largely something untrustworthily reported that happened long ago. Thanks, or no thanks, to the snapshot, we live in historical reality from the moment we are old enough to look at a Polaroid picture taken two minutes ago.
>
> Willingly or unwillingly, we are participating in a revolution in seeing which began when the first snapshots were taken about a hundred years ago. Call it, for want of a better phrase, the democratization of vision. (p. 108)

Although we seldom think of a mirror as a causal agent, it seems apparent that the ubiquitous snapshot has both mirrored and influenced our Western culture, as both the culture and photography have evolved together during the 20th century. It was perhaps only natural, therefore, that such an important, if sometimes invisible, influence on inner- and inter-personal relationships should become an increasingly significant component in psychotherapy.

USE OF SNAPSHOTS IN THERAPY

"On Christmas mornings my father was a photographer." Thus begins Papageorge's (1974, p. 24) description of what had become an annual family ritual, echoed in countless homes throughout the industrialized world. This festive aspect of "snapshooting" is so common that it is almost overlooked, yet it is one of the most positive attributes that photography can utilize in therapeutic settings. The vast majority of snapshots are the product of the interaction of people during happy occasions, positive experiences, or festive events. Although the same relatives may gather for other significant family events, generally more snapshots are taken at the weddings than at the funerals.

The introduction of photography into a therapeutic setting therefore has the potential to induce initial positive responses on the part of clients, even before a photographic activity is undertaken. It is a common cultural activity — as contrasted, for example, with group therapy — and snapshooting has few aesthetic overtones. It is not an act for which the participant will normally be judged, for it is an activity in which no one feels either heavily invested nor totally responsible. As Craven (1975) states,

> Today snapshots, with all their charm, are the most common and innocent examples of this fundamental approach. Common, of course, because they are produced by the millions, and innocent because a person taking a snapshot typically is most conscious of what happens to be in front of his camera, and least aware, at that moment, of the photograph which will result. That photograph, and everything it contains and means, are discovered later when he sees the print. (p. 124)

This lack of aesthetic criticism of snapshots can be a positive feature for the phototherapist, as it removes the judgmental component from the counseling process, a process that does not need that aesthetic judgment of 1000 years of Western art or 140 years of photography impacting on what is already a very tenuous balance.

There are several other qualities that make the snapshot useful in a therapeutic setting: the image is relatively inexpensive, it is lightweight and eminently portable, and it is very transformable, allowing it to be physically made into and combined with many other things, from T-shirts to collages.

It is also apparent that the effectiveness of the current therapeutic use of snapshots, in all of their idiosyncratic manifestations, is the result of the technical photographic breakthrough in the late 1880s. The inexpensive amateur camera and the resultant snapshots suddenly presented families and individuals with a multitude of pictorial artifacts that were both confirmations of, and confrontations with, their behaviors, relationships, and above all, their unique individuality. Ironically, it is the very proliferation of these and other visual images into our daily lives that has made us so blissfully unaware of their influence.

Elliott, in his essay introduction to *Dorothea Lange* (1966), reminds us that "In every art, glancing is an enemy of vision, but in none so much as in photography" (p. 6). The combining of photography's unique property of minute recording of detail with its facility as a pervasive and infinitely repeatable advertising and communications medium has resulted in a cultural desensitization to all but the most graphically potent images. As a result, the mental health practitioner who wishes to make maximum therapeutic use of photographic images must frequently learn new ways of seeing — i.e. reading — photographs, if the many nuances available through a patient viewing process are to be discovered.

As Newhall (1949) points out, "Camera pictures have been made ever since the Renaissance" (p. 9). With the assistance of such devices as the 'camera obscura,' artists had already developed a pictorial and spatial representation system based on a vanishing point perspective prior to Daguerre's announcement in 1839 of his method for permanently capturing the elusive camera obscura image. Thus, with the invention of photography, the artist, the photographic image, and the human eye were all viewing the world from a similar perspective, a perspective that places the viewer at the center of an optical universe.

Maholy-Nagy (1969) defines photography as "the visual presentation of what can be optically apprehended" (p. 39). The function of that visual presentation is expanded by Kozloff (1974) when he states that "with photography, we have concrete proof that we have not been hallucinating all our lives" (p. 64). Such an awareness of the conceptual role played by the photographic image, however, came much later in the development of photographic history, for earlier concerns were primarily with the visual and technical aspects of the medium.

According to Craven (1975),

> A photograph, however strong its resemblance to actual objects or events, does not accurately mirror the world. Nor does it show things as we see them. These differences between the way things appear to us and to the camera are not imaginary: they are very real. (p. 64)

Craven went on to enumerate the differences between retinal and film reception of light, the binocular human vision as opposed to the monocular vision of the camera, and the human reception of a continuous color spectral range as compared with film's recording of black-and-white or three primary colors.

Craven (1975) also pointed out that whereas the camera sees an entire scene at once and indiscriminately, we humans see more slowly and selectively, building a montage of visual impressions until we have mentally "assembled" the entire scene. This process establishes the basis for the self-statement aspect of photographic images, for according to Craven (1975),

> We see largely what we want to see, what our mind allows us to see, and even that constantly changes. Here, then, enter our personal concerns, our prejudices, our opinions — in other words, our whole system of human values. These, of course, differ for each one of us. All affect what we see, and therefore no two individuals see the same. (p. 6)

Additionally, any consideration of photography must continually take into account several dualities inherent in the medium: (a) the sometimes conflicting demands of *form* and *content,* (b) the likelihood that an image may be *of* one thing but *about* something else, (c) the fact that the photograph is both a *physical object* and an impression or *illusion* of something else, and (d) the awareness that the image is both *optical* and *conceptual.* It is the tensions generated by these dichotomies that give the medium its power while at the same time leading to perceptual confusions and ambiguities. Maholy-Nagy (1969), a leading figure in the twentieth century's exploration of the photographic image, discusses the issue of the photographic optical-conceptual relationship:

> We have hitherto used the capacities of the camera in a secondary sense only. This is apparent too in the so-called "faulty" photographs: the view from above, from below, the oblique view, which today often disconcert people who take them to be accidental shots. The secret of their effect is that the photographic camera reproduces the purely optical image and therefore shows the optically true distortions, deformations, foreshortenings, etc., whereas the eye together with our intellectual experience, supplements perceived optical phenomena by means of association and formally and spatially creates a *conceptual image.* Thus in the photographic camera we have the most reliable aid to a beginning of objective vision. (p. 28)

Arnheim (1957) points out that the mind not only is capable of making perceptual adjustments in form, but that it does the same thing with time and space when we are confronted with a series of photographic images, be they still or motion pictures:

> In real life every experience or chain of experiences is enacted for every observer in an uninterrupted spatial and temporal sequence. . . . There are no jerks in time or space in real life. Time and space are continuous. Not so in film. The period of time that is being photographed may be interrupted at any point. . . . And the continuity of space may be broken in the same manner. (pp. 20-21)

This freedom to manipulate time and space gives the photographer the opportunity to create individual responses to the perceived environment; i.e. to engage in personal expression. The ability to create new visual forms and concepts is enhanced by the camera's ability to make visible events in both time and space that are not available to the unaided human eye, and thus not perceived in the mind: the articulated golfer's swing, the time-compressed blooming of a rose, the close-up of a Jovian moon. Frampton (1974) claims that both angels and devils reside not so much in space, but in time — and that the camera can search them out in both places.

From the foregoing, it is evident that "seeing" is not an automatic function of the human eye, but is rather a conceptual image formed by the mind. It is based on the optical image formed on the retina, but it is in no way an exact duplication of that image. Berenson (1948) reinforces the old observation that "I wouldn't have seen it if I hadn't believed it with my own mind," when he states:

> We must discard the notion that photography reproduces an object as it is, as the objective 'itness' of anything. There is no such thing. The average man supposes that if the camera gives him an image of a thing corresponding to his own way of seeing it, that image is an exact, albeit two-dimensional, reduced and colorless counterfeit. He has never been told that his way of seeing has a long history behind it, utilitarian, practical, cannibal even. He takes it for granted that he sees 'reality,' that is to say something outside himself, corresponding exactly to what he sees. Seeing is as much an acquired art as speaking, although no doubt easier to learn. (p. 220)

Berenson's observation points out for the phototherapist the area of potential discrepancies between what the therapist "sees" in a photograph and what the client "sees" in the same image. He also makes additionally clear the cautions necessary in interpreting client photographs outside the presence of the client. For ultimately it is the client who actively makes the image fit his version of reality and creates its meaning.

Frampton (1974) postulated that the invention of photography has allowed us to celebrate "the moment of perception" as separate from all other moments (p. 45); i.e. prior to photography, our concept of time was that of a continuum from which *events* might be singled out, but seldom *moments*. Kozloff (1974) examines the relationship between photography and memory, when he states:

> Though infested with many bewildering anomalies, photographs are considered our best arbiters between our visual perceptions and our memories of them. It is not only their apparent "objectivity" that grants photographs their high status in this regard, but our belief that in them, fugitive sensation has been laid to rest. (p. 64)

According to Kozloff (1974), this has only occurred subsequent to the invention of photography, since "Painting and drawing, obviously, seldom get construed in this fashion because their relationship to the world is entirely hypothetical" (p. 65). It apparently requires at least the impression of objectivity engendered by the photographic image in order to engage our temporal sense of immediacy in activities and events.

The neurological studies of the brain's apparent lateral hemisphere specialization by Sperry, Bogen, Vogel, Gazzaniga, and others (Ornstein, 1977) seem to indicate that a good bit of the visual integrative functioning in activities such as photography, and the conceptualization that occurs during the viewing of the resultant images, occurs in the right hemisphere of most human brains. In a culture that has traditionally favored the left hemisphere with an emphasis upon rationality, sequencing, and analysis (Sagan, 1974), the rapid increase in visually related activities may ultimately have a physical effect on the expansion of right-hemisphere size, capacity, and functioning. Should this be the case, visual perception would apparently play an even more central role in our individual and cultural development.

Arnheim (1957) offers a possible relationship between the concept of the evolutionary development of our triune brain — the reptilian complex, limbic system, and neocortex (Sagan, 1977) and the emotional impact that the visual image can produce, as well as the dominance of the visual image when it and a verbal concept are perceived simultaneously:

> Sound and image are primordial art, closer to nature than the rendering by concepts. Music, painting, sculpture, architecture, dance, and film appeal to the more primitive side of the human mind. Although enlightened by speech, man nevertheless cherishes these ancient resources and their vigorously simple interpretation of what he has to say.
>
> Being more concrete and biologically older, the image can produce the more massive effects, so that the word is threatened when the picture, and particularly the moving picture, presents itself. (p. 218)

It might therefore be speculated that the use of visual images in phototherapy may facilitate therapeutic contact with deeper areas of client emotions, than those that are available to language and verbal concepts.

Maholy-Nagy (1957) believed that the advent of multi-media communications, as well as the polyphonic and polyoptical environments of contemporary urban cultures, had already initiated a change in our perceptive patterns. He contends that, "We have — through a hundred years of photography and two decades of film — been enormously enriched in this respect. We may say that we see the world with entirely different eyes" (p. 29)

In terms of the use of client photographs as self-statements in phototherapy, the way clients see the world has been conditioned by the photograph, and the way clients make or see photographs is conditioned by their world.

Summary

This chapter has looked at the development of photography as a pervasive influence in contemporary culture, and how it has changed the way we see and understand the world. It has attempted to bring to light characteristics and concerns of the medium as discussed by photographers, writers and critics. It has sought to show how the personal and projective quality of the simple snapshot, which forms the mainstay of phototherapy stimulus material, is a rich resource. This resource can be utilized in the therapeutic session to explore client concerns and their perceptions of themselves and the world. Finally, this chapter has stressed the importance of a therapist's ability to explore these images with clients so that the process is approached knowledgeably. This allows clients to become aware of the symbols of their own making, so that they may better understand their way of being in the world. By considering the history of the medium of photography in this context it is hoped that the reader will have a more broadly based understanding of some of the inherent commonalities in personal photography and psychotherapy, and how these commonalities led to the development of the field of phototherapy.

REFERENCES

Arbus, D. *Diane Arbus.* Millerton, N.Y.: Aperture, Inc., 1972.

Arnheim, R. *Film as art.* Berkeley: University of California Press, 1957.

Berenson, B. *Aesthetics and history.* Garden City, N.Y.: Doubleday & Company, Inc., 1954.

Bunnell, P. Taken from life. In D.P. Vanderlip (Ed.), *Photographic portraits.* Philadelphia: Moore College of Art, 1972.

Byers, P. Camera don't take pictures. *Columbia University Forum,* 1966, *9*(1), 27-32.

Craven, G.M. *Object and image.* Englewood Cliffs, N.J.: Prentice-Hall, Inc., 1975.

Elliott, G.P. On Dorothea Lange. In *Dorothea Lange.* New York: The Museum of Modern Art, 1966.

Frampton, H. Incisions in history/segments of eternity. *Artforum,* 1974, *13*(2), 39-50.

Sigmund Freud-house catalogue. Vienna, Austria: Sigmund-Freud Gesellschaft, 1975.

Friedlander, L. *Self portrait.* New City, N.Y.: Haywire Press, 1970.

Gernsheim, H. *A concise history of photography.* New York: Grosset & Dunlap, 1965.

Green, J. (Ed.). *The snapshot.* Millerton, N.Y.: Aperture, Inc., 1974.

Gilman, S. (Ed.). *The face of madness.* Secaucus, N.J.: Citadel Press, 1976.

Hall, J.B. Biographical essay. In M. Hoffman (Ed.), *Minor White: Rites and Passages.* Millerton, N.Y.: Aperture, Inc., 1978.

Hattersley, R. *Discover your self through photography.* New York: Association Press, 1971.

Hattersley, R. Introduction. In D. White, *Of women — of self.* Richmond, Va: author, 1977.

Hill, P., & Cooper, T. *Dialogue with photography.* New York: Farrar/Strauss/Giroux, 1979.

Hoffman, M. (Ed.). *Minor White: Rites and Passages.* Millerton, N.Y.: Aperture, Inc., 1978.

Jacobs, D.L. Portraits of the artists. *Afterimage,* 1979, *7*(1 & 2), 17-18.

Jung, C.G. (Ed.). *Man and his symbols.* London, England: Aldus Books Limited, 1964.

Kemp, W.D. *Photography for visual communicators.* New York: Prentice-Hall, Inc., 1973.

Kouwenhoven, J.A. Essay. In J. Green (Ed.), *The snapshot.* Millerton, N.Y.: Aperture, Inc., 1974.

Kozloff, M. The territory of photographs. *Artforum,* 1974, *13*(3), 64-67.

Krauss, D. *The uses of still photography in counseling and therapy: Development of a training model.* Unpublished doctoral dissertation, Kent State University, 1979.

Lesy, M. Snapshots: Psychological documents, frozen dreams. *After-image,* 1976, *4*(4), 12-13.

Lyons, N. (Ed.). *Photographers on photography.* Englewood Cliffs, N.J.: Prentice-Hall., 1966.

MacNeil, W.S. Essay and photographs. In J. Green (Ed.), *The snapshot.* Millerton, N.Y.: Aperture, Inc., 1974.

Maholy-Nagy, L. *Painting, photography, film.* Cambridge, Mass.: The MIT Press, 1969. (Originally published, 1925).

Model, L. Essay and photographs. In J. Green (Ed.), *The snapshot.* Millerton, N.Y.: Aperture, Inc., 1974.

Newhall, B. *The history of photography.* New York: The Museum of Modern Art, 1949.

Norman, D. *Alfred Stieglitz: An American seer.* Millerton, N.Y.: Aperture, Inc., 1973.

Ornstein, R.E. *The psychology of consciousness* (2nd ed.). New York: Harcourt Brace Jovanovich, Inc., 1977.

Papageorge, T. Essay and photographs. In J. Green (Ed.), *The snapshot.* Millerton, N.Y.: Aperture, Inc., 1974.

Phillips, D. Viewpoints. *Photo Ovo,* 1975, Jan./Feb. (19), 7.

Sagan, C. *The dragons of Eden.* New York: Random House, 1977.

Shortenwyde, R.J. *Photography as huckster.* Tupelo, Miss.: Rambling Press, 1943.

Sontag, S. *On photography.* New York: Farrar, Strauss and Giroux, 1977.

Stewart, D. Photo therapy: Theory and practice. *Art Psychotherapy, 6*(1), 41-46. (a)

Stewart, D. Photo therapy comes of age. *Kansas Quarterly,* 1979, *11*(4), 19-46, (b)

Stieglitz, A. How I came to photograph clouds. In N. Lyons (Ed.) *Photographers on photography.* Englewood Cliffs, N.J.: Prentice-Hall, Inc., 1966. (Reprinted from *The amateur photographer & photography.* 1923, *56*(1819), 225.)

Sturr, E. Introduction. *Kansas Quarterly,* Fall 1979*, 11,*(4)5.

Szarkowski, J. (Ed.). *E.J. Bellocq: Storyville portraits.* New York: The Museum of Modern Art, 1970.

Upton, B., and Upton, J. *Photography.* Boston: Little, Brown and Company, 1976.

White, M. What is meant by "reading" photographs. *Aperture,* 1957, *5*(2), 48-50.

White, M. Equivalence: The perennial trend. In N. Lyon (ed.), *Photographers on Photography.* Englewood Cliffs, N.J.: Prentice-Hall, Inc., 1966. (Reprinted from *PSA Journal,* 1963, *29* (7), 17-21.)

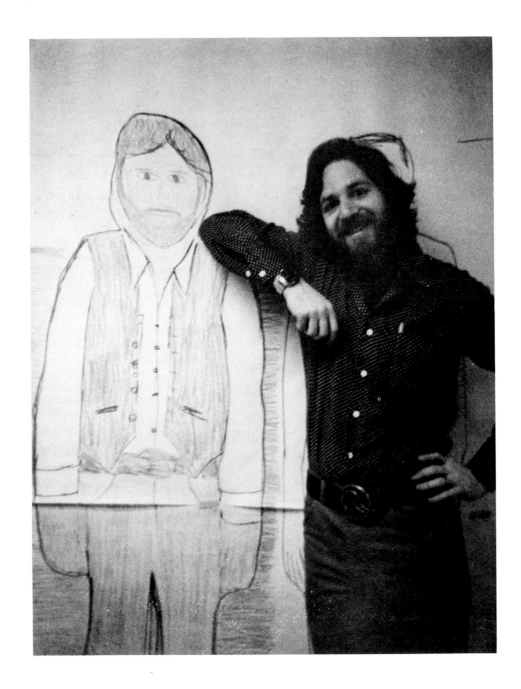

Photo by Anne M. Gatti

Chapter 3

Reality, Photography and Psychotherapy

All through history, man has searched for ultimate reality by various means, mystical and intuitive, rational and scientific. Today, some thousands of years after the launching of this search, we have had to throw up our hands with Einstein and modern philosophy and declare that all is relative to our perceptual equipment and to our transcendent place. (Becker, 1971, p. 190)

HISTORICAL REVIEW

SINCE the earliest human beings first became aware of themselves, each a unique "I," alone, in a mysterious and powerful universe; since they first became aware of their ephemeral existence on this physical world, people have been concerned with and preoccupied by understanding the nature of reality. This has been especially clear since the time of Plato and the Greek philosophers. Both learned and simple people alike have sought to discover what is real, what is not. In the twentieth century, however, the questions about the nature of reality have entered our lives at an accelerated pace. We live in a technologically sophisticated world, we have more scientific data about our own and other universes and yet, ironically, we discover that the nature of reality may always remain a mystery, just out of our reach.

It is in the twentieth century that the most radical concepts in the arts and sciences have found their way into our lives. These include Planck's quantum theory (1900), Freud's interpretation of dreams (1905), the advent of Cubism (1907), Einstein's theory of relativity (1908), and the advent of abstract painting (1910). Although over seventy-five years old, these concepts and new ideas in arts and sciences influenced by these concepts affect our lives, our civilization, and our personal and collective consciousness daily. Whereas once it was not unusual for western people to believe that the laws for moral behavior were universal and absolute, they are now exposed to the conceptual ideas of "cultural relativity" and "situational ethics." Whereas once people believed they could truly know themselves, they are now told that two-thirds of their consciousness, i.e. their very existence, is out of reach, unconscious, perhaps unknowable. Whereas once people walked the woods and knew a tree to be a

41

tree, solid and hard, firm and durable, now they are told it is molecular energy, constantly in motion. These advances in science and art have shattered whatever concept of an absolute reality people once held and have created the uncertainty of knowing appearance is not reality.

The field and practice of psychotherapy have flourished in this last half of the twentieth century. This, most surely, is related to the inevitable tensions and difficulties of being a human being in a world of flux. As thinking, feeling and acting beings, we have the mental capability to know well our tenuous position in the universe. Likewise, we know well that there is much that we can never know: we are unable to answer large questions such as what exactly exists after death; and we cannot be assured of the correct way to live a life. Without tradition-bound limits and societal or cultural absolutes to guide and direct us, we are denied an easy life of acquiescence and safety. Conflicting facts continually confront us. We become confused. We are conflicted. We are psychologically unsure. With this in mind, it is easy to see why so many people enter into psychotherapy; they seek to establish or reestablish a structure or order, a meaning in their lives. They wish to expand, through experience, their personal awareness. Ideally, they hope to find a behavioral change while, realistically, most come to get reassurance for their neurosis. Most of all, they seek to relieve the pain of living in an age of uncertainty, during a time of transitions.

Contemporary phototherapy, as an emerging approach to psychotherapy, responds to the effects of accelerated change in our lives. It allows clients, and, in fact, encourages clients to examine their lives and to review their personal histories through the photobiographic use of snapshots and the family album. It also encourages clients to communicate photographically (visually) how they experience the world, both in the past and in the here and now, and to discover the important personal symbols they choose to express that experience: i.e. the meanings of people, places and things and themes that appear in their photos. It uses photos as a catalyst to address client concerns.

Phototherapy utilizes both symbolism and projection as the basic technique or tool for treatment. Photographs taken by clients concretely and symbolically portray objects that are directly related to their mental state and to their "map of reality." In other words, the photo has the ability to show actual objects as well as to symbolically present "I statements" (as in projective test materials). Therefore, the way clients personally make sense out of the vast number of stimuli that impinge upon their senses is at least partially represented or implied in every photograph. This map of reality is a symbolic representational system constructed from the elements of physiology, socialization, and personal experience. It allows humans to believe that they understand the world they live in by defining the paradigms by which they experience it. For instance, photographs taken by a client or drawn from the family album offer examples of the ways the world is defined, represented, and remembered by the individual. Photographs not only record a point of view, they also encourage the maintenance of that point of view in memory and imply a mindset. Photographic images reveal a metaphoric map that relates to one's participation in life; they may range from the extremes of a narrow and constricting viewpoint to a lack of structure or boundaries of any type. These maps represented in the photographs are different for every individual, and we must first consider where they come from before we can move therapeutically to help clients change them to be more functional. Let us first consider the components of this map: Biology, socialization, and personal experience.

COMPONENTS OF THE MAP OF REALITY:
BIOLOGICAL BASIS FOR PERCEPTION

Earlier in this chapter several lines were drawn from sociologist Ernest Becker (1971), "all is relative to our perceptual equipment and transcendent place" (p. 190). People's perceptual equipment is determined, shaped and limited by our unique biological make-up. It is the utilization of our biological sensory apparatus which allows us to receive and order the vast amount of internal and external stimuli which constantly bombards us. Our ability to taste, touch, smell, hear and see permits us to orient ourselves to the world.

It is clear that physiologically we human beings experience the world in a very incomplete way. In fact, much of what we call technology exists to compensate for sense deficit. Our senses, the foundation by which we experience, order and prioritize stimuli, can gather only limited information about the world, i.e. there are finite limits to the kind of and amount of information that our senses can access. For example, our visual sense does not let us see the infrared or ultraviolet portions of the spectrum. (We create the ontological rationalization that we see the "visible spectrum" of light.) We have neither the precise distance vision of the eagle or the refined night vision of the owl. Our auditory sense does not have the capacity to hear high frequencies audible to canines or many other animals. Kinesthetically, while our heads, hands and feet are relatively sensitive to touch, to air and to temperature gradation, areas of our backs are not. Many times our sense of balance and gyroscopic orientation to the world leaves much to be desired. Other animals are certainly more finely tuned kinesthetically. Our olfactory and gustatory senses are also limited. Although all of our senses can be developed and refined, there seem to be certain finite limitations placed upon our sensory apparatus as a part of physiological wiring of the organism.

Not only does there seem to be finite limits to the kind and amount of information that our senses can access, also it seems that this accessing can only take place in specialized areas of the brain, as research in hemispherical differentiation has documented. This is mentioned here because the "dominant" brain hemisphere is a determining factor in the biological basis for perception.

The left-brain dominant (logical and linear) way of accessing and representing reality seems to be very different from the right-brain dominant (intuitive and nonlinear) way of assessing and representing reality. Hemispherical dominance determines how and which senses will be utilized in accepting, processing and utilizing data. Since our culture is predominantly left hemispherically dominant, clients who have right-brain hemispherical dominance may experience language and/or communication problems. Working with these clients phototherapeutically validates their personal experience of the world and allows them to experience techniques by which they may make a transition into understanding the world in different ways.

In addition to these initial limitations inherent in the species, we are biologically set up to select, disregard, and prioritize the vast amount of stimuli our system is programmed for and subjected to. For instance, we tend to prioritize, and hence perceive, a moving object more quickly than a stationary object. Clearly this was an essential skill to develop at an early point in the evolution of the species for the moving object could spell either sustenance or danger. It was essential for humankind's survival that such a stimulus became a priority of perception. A second example of a biological hierarchy of perception can be discerned when our physiological need for food governs our perception of objects in a room. When hungry, what we notice is that which will satisfy our hunger, not a new book, or a painting, or the letters on the desk. In this sense then, we are groomed to differentiate a given perceptual field. From a gestalt framework, we may say that we experience (see, feel, intuit, think) a primary figure emerging from a ground. In a general sense, this biological perspective allows us to differentiate and, hence, perceive objects in the environment.

Since our senses are our first link with the world, it follows that the more we can utilize any and/or all of our sensory inputs at any given time (up to the point of sensory overload), the more information we have to work with in choosing how to respond to the world. This gives us more options for behaving. The ability to fluidly utilize any one or combination of senses and to translate that sensory input into information and action increases our chances for a more appropriate and successful response to the environment and increases our chances for survival. Having a number of options available for responding to the environment is not unrelated to certain concepts of evolution. Since the engagement of any sensory mode entails a disregarding of information from other sensory channels, some of our ability to functionally employ all of our senses may greatly diminish over time. It is in this area where psychotherapists and counselors can work with clients to help them reclaim their ability to make contact with themselves and the world by developing and enlarging their sensory orientations.

This implies in a larger sense, that effective mental health professionals should be able to utilize all of *their* senses in their professional settings. (This has broad implications for professional training). Mental health professionals, therefore, are most effective when they are able to read sensory orientation cues and to make contact with the client regardless of that client's dominant sensory orientation to the world. They are then prepared, by using a client's primary sensory orientation as a base, to help the client translate his or her experience into different sense channels so that the experience can be accessed and represented differently. As we will see when we examine the phototherapeutic applications of the visual sense orientation, this allows clients to increase and enhance sensory input and awareness, and can positively influence their resultant behaviors.

COMPONENTS OF THE MAP OF REALITY:
SOCIOLOGICAL AND INDIVIDUAL BASIS FOR PERCEPTION

Our map of reality is more than biological; it is also influenced and partially determined by our cultural perspective and individual experience. Living in any culture teaches us a great deal about how we "should" experience the world. This "should" influences what we attend to and/or disregard in our environment; this is the process of socialization. Through this process, we learn what is deemed acceptable and what is unacceptable, what is real and what is not, and how the real may be experienced and understood. Socialization, thus, involves the teaching of a specific orientation about "how to be" in the world. Responses to this being in the world are evident in different cultures' diverse orientations to the individual, the family, childrearing, choosing a mate, work, and so forth. It also manifests itself within a culture in terms of class structure that allows certain life opportunities and options for some and not for others. Socialization is also the teaching of "that's the way it is."

Socialization provides a powerful answer to the question, "What is real?" What is real is the mutually shared explanation of the world, passed on through generations in any given culture. Although learning about the world is clearly essential for the young child trying to orient himself/herself in a mysterious world of wonder, there are some serious shortcomings inherent in the socialization process, as mentioned by Gregory Bateson (1972) in *Steps to an Ecology of Mind,* and Grinder and Bandler (1975) in *The Structure of Magic* (volumes I and II). As each author observed, individuals too often fail to realize that their personal-cultural map that represents reality is nothing more than that, a personal-cultural map. Too often, this map is taken for reality itself. Its unique symbolic shorthand is no longer understood metaphorically. The danger in believing this fallacy is that we not only lose our ability to imagine and, hence, create alternative innovative maps of reality, but that we may also become caught up in a struggle to perpetuate a map that is long out of date. The history of civilization is full of such examples, which include: ideas of a flat world, the sun moving around the earth, witchcraft trials, concepts of a master race, or atoms as the smallest particles of matter. Humankind continually wages a psychic war to maintain the belief that a cultural map of reality is reality itself.

The implication of this line of thought is that a shared and universal reality is both naive and impossible. That which we deem real is nothing other than a perception of reality limited by our perceptual equipment aided by whatever technology we have available. We have seen that these perceptions are determined by our biology, our social-cultural indoctrination, and our individual experience in the world. Together, these components compose our perceptual set, the system we use to find and choose our map of reality. Reality can thus be viewed as existential or phenomenological. That is to say that the reality of any event lies in the ability of the perceiver to perceive it as an event and to integrate it into his/her schema for being in the world. Furthermore, if a stimulus cannot be incorporated into the perceptual field, it is not a part of our reality. (For a detailed explanation and exploration of this position, see Combs, Richards, & Richards, 1976, *Perceptual Psychology*; and Segall, Campbell, & Herskovitz, 1966, *The Influence of Culture on Visual Perception.*)

In this regard, one is reminded of the ancient story of the three blind men and the elephant. As one rendition of the story states:

> Beyond Ghor there was a city. All its inhabitants were blind. A king with his entourage arrived nearby; he brought his army and camped in the desert. He had a mighty elephant which he used in attack and to increase the people's awe.
>
> The populace became anxious to learn about the elephant, and some sightless from among this blind community ran like fools to find it. Since they did not know even the form or shape of the elephant, they groped sightlessly, gathering information by touching some part of it. Each thought that he knew something, because he could feel a part.
>
> When they returned to their fellow citizens, eager groups clustered around them, anxious, misguidedly, to learn the truth from those who were themselves astray. They asked about the form, the shape of the elephant, and they listened to all they were told.
>
> The man whose hand had reached an ear said: "It is a large rough thing, wide and broad like a rug."
>
> One who felt the trunk said: "I have the real facts about it. It is like a straight and hollow pipe, awful and destructive."
>
> One who had felt its feet and legs said: "It is might and firm, like a pillar."
>
> Each had felt one part out of the many. Each had perceived it wrongly. No mind knew all: knowledge is not the companion of the blind. All imagined something, something incorrect. The created is not informed about divinity. There is no way in this science by means of the ordinary intellect. (Ornstein, 1972, pp. 161-162)

Reality, like the multitudinous parts of the elephant, cannot be easily known or perceived piecemeal. The average person today, perhaps all persons always, are in the situation of the blind men in this tale. They know only what their senses allow them to perceive. They know only their limited subjective experience and, most importantly, that which they know may well be a different reality from their fellow blind men, their neighbors. Later in this book we will learn how phototherapy explores and expands client realities.

CREATION OF MEANING

We have seen that our personal experience of the world comes about via the assessing of incoming information that is transmitted through our senses to the brain, where it is organized, given meaning and represented. This experiencing is derived and dependent on our biology, socialization, and individual experience, which creates sensory orientation to the world. We have seen that we cannot directly experience the world, but have to experience it through our senses. The process of organizing and making sense out of the vast amount of input we receive through our senses is a process of the representation of reality through symbology. These symbols, by definition, have meanings and associations that are larger than any one object, element, or relationship. There exists a vast literature concerning the nature and function of symbolism which is exemplified in writings of Combs et al. (1976), Hall (1959), Jung (1964), Reusch (1969), and many others. In this section, I will identify, review, and give examples of the most pertinent symbolic processes as they bear on our larger discussion.

First of all, we know that the symbolizing process takes place at both the aware and unaware level of consciousness, and that each of these levels affects the other. On the primarily conscious level, we can look at perception as a product of symbolizing. For example, our eyes sense a figure emerging from a ground: a tree in a meadow. The light reflected from the figural tree is taken in by the eye via the retina, and is transmitted to the brain by the optic nerve. The neural impulses are received by the brain in a specific area where they are reassembled and translated into the image of a tree where, in combination with other information, it is given signficance. Just exactly how the tree is "seen" is dependent on the cultural and personal meanings surrounding it. The tree's meaning is a result of its learned context and is an example of the symbolizing process, for the tree represents more to us than its physically discerned properties. It might be viewed as a hiding place, a shelter, a source of nourishment in the form of fruit, a place where people are hanged, a source of building supplies, or a sacred place, etc. The symbolizing process takes objects from the world, combines them with contexts, and endows them with deeper and/or broader meanings.

Let us for a moment consider these typed words themselves. How do they derive their meaning? Their meaning derives from our ability to cause them to make sense. It is possible to view them simply as a random way to put ink on a page and consequently seek no further meaning. They may be seen as some sort of graphic pattern, or more complexly as a systematic way of putting ink on a page. They may be further differentiated and grouped as letters, words, phrases, sentences, and paragraphs that will have a generally agreed upon meaning by sighted readers of English. We come to this general agreement through the utilization of our biological inheritance and the symbols we have learned as a result of our socialization and individual experience.

The meaning of writing is more than the words. Even if one who did not speak English had access to a dictionary that translated English words into this person's native tongue, he or she would still not understand idiomatic meanings and associations (symbolic) which merge from the combining of words and phrases. On the conscious level this is sometimes referred to as being able to read between the lines. These written words are part of a conscious and explicit symbol system that the culture shares. Needless to say, this agreed upon meaning is artificial and would not exist for anyone who could not read English. It would be outside of their reality because they did not have the symbols or the context to incorporate it into their map of the world. Obviously many things exist in the world that are outside of the reality of those who lack the sense orientation to access them or the context in which to place them. The unexperienced phenomena become part of the undifferentiated ground from which figural areas emerge and become dominant.

There is a constant interplay of influences on, and no clearcut distinction between, conscious and unconscious symbols. Arnheim (1971), in *Visual Thinking,* states that even Freudian symbolism which is based on concerns with the reproductive organs is not based on their attributes *per se*, but rather is abstracted or distilled from concepts of shape or function. In other words, unconscious symbols share the same process of formulation as do conscious symbols; the product of unconscious symbols is simply out of our awareness. Both conscious and unconscious symbols seek to represent our needs and perceived relationship to the world. Unconscious symbols may simply be more spontaneous or less censored by the socialization process.

Clearly the influence on conscious and unconscious symbol system by socialization and enculturation is enormous. The fields of visual anthropology and visual sociology study these phenomena on an ongoing basis in order to more clearly perceive the nature of these processes and their effects from a societal point of view. Attitudes learned from the socialization process and our culture influence our perceptions of associations with objects, concepts, and places. There are certain advantages to sharing a common map with symbols we hold in common. On the surface, it allows us to go about our daily lives in some semblance of relationship to others in our culture. However, worth and value are ascribed to certain symbols in a culture that alter an individual's map of reality. For example, if a fruit tree is seen as unapproachable because of a particular ascribed value, then the hungry individual will not be able to assuage his hunger. On a more internal process level, a rich source of potential experience may not be available. Socialization teaches us to incorporate as our own the agreed-upon cultural symbols that offer explanation for the world and, hence, devalue individual personal symbols. Schizophrenia is an extreme example of the devaluation of personal symbols by a culture. The paradox of this phenomenon is that the more we are socialized, thereby learning and accepting the cultural values and symbols, the more we lose our own internal symbol system; and, therefore, our unique and personal experience of the world is diminished.

We come to believe the symbols learned through socialization as our own organic symbols. The dangers of this are obvious from both an authentic personal and societal perspective. We know that evolution has always favored diversity and adaptability. All great breakthroughs in science and art have occurred because individuals have relied upon their personal symbol systems to the extent that they have transcended the existing culturally defined and limited paradigms. The history of civilization is one of creating new paradigms that advance the culture again. This has always been the task of artists and scientists.

There obviously needs to be a balance between individual and cultural symbols, for without such an arrangement, there would be no culture from which to evolve. These symbols are helpful to communicate ideas, feelings, and experiences. We cannot help but be influenced consciously and unconsciously by cultural symbols, and we must not underestimate their pervasiveness. In order that we have the option to incorporate our unique and personal view of the world onto our map of reality, it is necessary to maintain a "tentativeness of belief."

There seems to be some overlap and commonality between certain individual and cultural symbols. These symbols may be called universal or archetypical for they are not dependent on any particular pattern of socialization. They seem to evolve spontaneously from the human psyche itself as a response to life. Jung (1964) studied these common symbols, which he considered part of humankind's collective unconscious. The great similarity of beliefs about creation and other religious myths from diverse early cultures, as written about by Campbell (1972), Jung (1964), and Read (1965), present strong evidence in support of this thesis.

The individual personal unconscious symbol is generally not available to our normal awareness. We can, however, look at dreams, drawings, art, literature, and photographs for examples of these symbols at work. Dream symbols offer a classic example. Dreams occur in a special physiological state called REM sleep (rapid movement of the closed eye), which can be identified by emission of specific brain waves as monitored on laboratory equipment. Dreaming seems to be a process by which pertinent concerns play themselves out via an unconscious symbolic story. Dreams have been shown to be a rich source of symbolic data. These personal unconscious symbols are derived from and influenced by our entire life experience, and their meanings are derived from the dreamer's context of personal history and concerns in the world. Any dream object/symbol may represent a number of things, depending on the context of the specific dream. Our unconscious is too active and inventive for it to be otherwise. For example, a tree in a dream might symbolize any of the associations that we have previously mentioned. The dream symbol must always be regarded in context to the rest of the dream and the dreamer's life. (The same is true for drawings and photographs.) Finally, for a dream symbol to be useful to a person, it must be able to be acknowledged by that person. Brilliant symbolic analysis is mere intellectual exercise, useless if the person is blocked to the extent that symbolic message and the relationship to personal concerns cannot be understood. Photographs, like single moments extracted and preserved from dreams, serve the purpose of supplying the therapist with a vast amount of information that both client and therapist can examine together. This information can be used in a variety of ways. In phototherapy analysis of photographs is often a technique for making contact and gaining rapport with clients through dialogue which initially focuses on the symbols in the image and then moves its focus to the client. This results from the therapist sharing his or her observations, questions, feelings and hunches which emerge from looking at the photograph with the client. During this process clients often supply additional information and will also "correct" therapists' mistakes in analysis or interpretation. As a result of this process, clients have more awareness and a better understanding of their personal symbols.

Freud (1963) did pioneering work in the area of personal symbols as manifestations of subconscious activity, and made use of them in his dream work.

> We experience it (a dream) predominantly in visual images; feelings may be present too, and thoughts interwoven as well; the other senses may also experience something, but nonetheless it is predominantly a question of images. Part of the difficulty of giving an account of dreams is due to our having to translate these visual images into words. "I could draw it" a dreamer often says to us, "but I don't know how to say it." (Freud, 1963, p. 90)

Freud (1963) always maintained that all personal symbols were negative and regressive. He thought that they served as defense mechanisms by transforming unconscious wishes into something that could be accepted by a conscious ego without trauma. Jung (1954), unlike Freud (1963), let his patients who wished to do so draw their dreams, and he found the practice useful. It led him to conclude that personal symbols may be used in the regressive way that Freud postulated, but that, additionally, they may also be used in a positive manner, aiding insight and providing a structure from which new thinking, understanding, and communication can evolve. May (1964) also discussed the nature of symbolism and likewise concluded that personal symbols can be defensive and regressive, as well as progressive and expansive. They can provide insight necessary to create new realities. Symbols have the potential to integrate new experience and give it meaning. This position is in agreement with both gestalt dream work (Downing & Marmerstein, 1973; Perls, Hefferline, & Goodman, 1951; Zinker, 1971) psychodrama (Moreno, 1972), and art therapy (Naumberg, 1966).

Gestalt psychologists, rather than focusing on the symbolic aspects of the dream, assume that every part of the dream is the dreamer. Within the dream state, we project ourselves and every bit and piece of the dream is part of our alienated personality.

As with photographs or other art productions, dreams don't just *belong* to you, they are you. Each and every one of your dreams (or photographs) is an expression of an infinite array of conflicts, harmonies, contradictions, and associations which make you the person you are. Each of your dreams (or photographs), when treated as containing any element of projection may be used as a point of departure on an endless road to self-awareness. In a gestalt way, elements of photography and dream material, can serve as signposts along the road to personal awareness and healthier functioning. Some signposts are bright — clearly focused and appropriately illuminated; others are dull, uninteresting, out of focus, obscured or completely dark. All contain the potency to facilitate a more meaningful journey inward into the unknown and undiscovered regions of our innerselves. (Woldt, 1979)

As Read (1965) has stated:

It is only insofar as the artist establishes symbols for the representation of reality that mind, as a structure of thought, can take shape. The artist establishes these symbols by becoming conscious of new aspects of reality, and by representing his consciousness of these new aspects of reality in plastic or poetic images. (p. 53)

What we choose to focus on in our photos demonstrates the themes of our personal symbols. Therapeutic change enlarges our intelligence insofar as it changes our outlook and options for being. Stated another way, we can paraphrase Read by saying that all thoughts derives from integration of symbols for reality. Our personal symbols, therefore, are the very crux of our intelligence.

Freud (1938) did not understand this primacy of personal symbols in creating a person's awareness and orientation to the world in other dysfunctional ways. He did not fathom their creative and integrative potency, and chose to work in the verbal mode which is most easily defended because it is the most familiar. Many times, however, we experience and know more than we can say about an event in our lives. This is so because of the limitations of our learned verbal symbols. Our words are products of an artificial system of symbols which try to approximate our experience and total understanding. Words can never do this, no matter how concise or elegant they might be. Our most powerful symbols are our nonverbal symbols, for they are essentially the source of our consciousness.

All words come from transpositions of internal experience to personal symbols, to the external symbol of verbal communication, a translated translation. The same concept in audio or optical terms would be called a third generation product; that is, the succeeding reproduction of the original information. We know that in any translation or succeeding reproduction, some information is lost via deletion or distortion, which changes the message. The reader may remember playing the game of telephone as a child, and what happened to the message as it passed from person to person.

People who speak more than one language fluently know that it is necessary to learn to think (create symbols) in a new way in order to master the second language. They also know that some experiences or concepts simply do not translate because they are not part of the other language's symbol system. The second language may have no words or phrases that represent certain internal aspects of reality. Our concept of time as being past, present, and future makes it difficult to understand the Hopi Indian concept of time which is symbolized quite differently. Additionally, our ease and familiarity with our own language makes it easy for us to censor our own meanings by deletion and distortion as long as we function in the purely verbal mode.

It is the symbolic, the personal symbol, which is created as a response to stimulus, that gives us the clearest indication of what is occurring at the unconscious or unaware level. It is in working with these symbols as manifest in dreams, drawings, or photographs that we have access to a powerful tool for creating inroads to understanding personal concerns and to help change occur.

Phototherapy concerns itself with personal symbols as projected through the visual representational system and manifest in the form of photographic images. Photos are considered to be representations of a client's reality. This is true not only of images made by clients, or which include the client, but also of any image chosen by the client from magazines, etc. The meaning of any image will be dependent on the client's personal "vision." As stated earlier, this is a basis for work with all projective materials. Phototherapy is helpful in overcoming the initial problems of verbal censoring as it pays attention to the symbol as the message, and is not dependent on the client's skill as a verbal communicator to describe his or her reality. The client and therapist together work with the image. This, of course, does not avoid completely the aforementioned problems of distortion and deletion, but it does lessen the effect of such a process as we initially work with the nonverbal symbols present in the image.

Phototherapy, while still a growing field, has a strong methodological and theoretical link to the already established field of art psychotherapy. Art psychotherapy deals with clients' symbols as presented primarily through drawing. It might be mentioned that while art therapy clients might initially be reluctant to draw as a result of their feelings of drawing incompetency, almost everyone feels competent enough to point and shoot a simple camera.

According to Naumberg (1966), the process of art therapy is:

> . . . based on the recognition that man's fundamental thoughts and feelings are derived from the unconscious and often reach expression in images rather than in words. By means of pictorial projection, art therapy encourages a method of symbolic communication between patient and therapist. . . . By projecting interior images into exteriorized designs photographs art therapy crystalizes and fixes in lasting form the recollection of dreams and fantasies (or any other event) which otherwise would remain evanescent and might be quickly forgotten. . . . The art therapist does not interpret the symbolic art expression of his patient, but encourages the patient to discover for himself the meaning of his art projections photographs. (p. 2)

One of the shared aspects of both art therapy and phototherapy is that analysis of the images allows clients to discover their own concerns and meanings. Although both art therapy and phototherapy utilize the methodology of pictorial projection, it would seem initially that they do so in very different ways. Art therapy relies on a client's internal concerns to emerge from the unconscious through the process of a drawing, spontaneously produced by the client. External stimuli, light or content, need not be available at the time a client draws a picture for an image to appear in the drawing. For example, a client might draw a house which is clearly not visible in the room where the drawing is taking place. Photographs, on the other hand, will be taken at the place where the physical content actually exists. A photograph of a house will use as content some physical representation of a house. Since art therapy is dependent on externalized internal subjects and phototherapy is dependent on internalized external subjects, it appears as though they deal with different aspects of personal symbolism. We need to remember, however, that both are projections and symbolic representations of a client's reality. The use of a camera in this process simply makes the projection seem to us, as a result of our socialization, more accurate and real than other pictorial representation. Both, however, are simply symbolic approximations of reality. Both processes are useful in allowing clients to pictorially create, experience and benefit from learning their symbols as a way to know more about themselves in the present.

Probably a greater difference between these two techniques lies in the availability for utilization of personal and family photographs in phototherapy; i.e. family mapping, environmental, and chronological information. These pictures present the client and members of the family engaged in various activities, at various occasions, over time. These historical photos provide a rich source of projective and physical data that could not be obtained any other way. They provide background information about a client's relationship to the world outside of therapy.

Before continuing our discussion of the ways in which photographs are useful in counseling and therapy, it may be helpful to consider the photograph itself as an entity. A photograph is usually a piece of paper or plastic that has been chemically treated with an emulsion which, when exposed to light and processed correctly, will yield either a color or black and white image. We view that flat surface of a photograph as if it were three-dimensional, even though we have some awareness of it being flat and essentially two-dimensional; we intentionally "distort" our reality. We need to do this in order for the photograph to make sense visually and correspond to the way we see other objects in space. That is to say that as viewer, we project the photograph as a window on the world and give it perspective, depth, and dimension according to our experience. Furthermore, this projection is an active process and does not happen automatically. Seeing the flat surface of a photograph as three-dimensional is a learned skill.

We also project certain gestalt laws of visual perception, as demonstrated by

Wertheimer in the early part of this century. Zakia's (1975) recent book, *Perception and Photography*, contains an excellent review of these principles. These laws include principles of figure-ground (where part of an image is seen as separate and standing out from a background), closure (where closed or complete visual elements are seen as figure), proximity (where the closer two or more visual elements appear to be, the greater their likelihood of being considered a group or pattern), and similarity (where visual images that are similar in size, shape, or color tend to be seen as related). All of these laws deal with the purely visual patterns of photographic content or other pictorial content, and help to explain why we perceive the way we do.

Photographs, however, are more than visual patterns that make up a content that can be described by gestalt laws. Additionally, they can be considered in terms such as abstract or concrete, static or dynamic, formal or informal, spontaneous or posed, active or passive, intuitive or contemplated, and so forth. A photograph may have all of the above characteristics in various degrees at any one time. This part of the content further supplies a context from which meaning can evolve.

In looking at the complexity and abundance of information that a photograph presents, the task of assigning a meaning to a photograph would be impossible without the benefits of shared symbolism. As mentioned earlier, it is through the process of socialization that we have available for our use a basic vocabulary of shared symbols, some of which seem to be universal. It is from this shared symbolism that we draw our basic vocabulary, which we modify and communicate in terms of our individual experience. Therefore, in viewing photographs, we are in the position of receiving messages (visual projections) that indicate how a client/photographer makes sense out of what he/she experiences and, even more fundamentally, what is that segment of the environment that is chosen to be represented.

In counseling and therapy, photographs may also provide evidence of a reality that the client is "blind to" for some reason. This might be the case when a client's report of a photograph's content or meaning are very different from what the photograph reveals to others. Photographs can then be used as confrontation devices that push clients to reexamine their perception in certain areas of their lives. Akeret (1973), in his book, *Photoanalysis,* discusses this technique in conjunction with several cases. Additionally and more generally, photographs help define and serve to focus on client issues. When a number of photographs by or of the same person are viewed sequentially, certain patterns or themes will emerge. In therapy, these themes can be starting points from which a client can be aided in working on areas that have been tentatively diagnosed through the joint viewing and discussion of photographs. It should be understood that as counselors and therapists who view and work with client photographs, we are aware and able to separate our personal themes from those of our clients, so that in working with a client's photo image, it remains as undistorted a process as possible.

Summary

In order to give the reader a background for understanding why phototherapy is a useful adjunctive therapeutic technique with a wide variety of practical applications, this chapter focused on a number of fundamental assumptions regarding the individual's process of creating personal meaning in the world. We considered certain aspects of biology as they pertained to our sensory apparatus; we considered the socialization process as a strong determinant in perceiving and valuing experience, and we considered the unique personal history of each person as it relates to his ability to create meaning in the here and now. The three areas of our discussion form the foundation of a human's outlook and point of view.

In the section devoted to biological determinants we noted that our senses, even as highly developed as they might be, only provide a certain amount of information. Our senses are our link with the world, and there is much of the world we live in that is beyond our experience because of the physiological limits of our sensory apparatus. Additionally we subjectively create favored patterns for the accessing and representation of our reality. We learn to select and prioritize information by creating unique individual maps of reality. These maps define the parameters by which we make the world make sense for us and are intrinsically tied to the socialization process which assigns value to experience by teaching us what is important to be aware of and what may be disregarded.

Much of this map exists outside of our awareness and is represented symbolically. These symbols emerge by endowing objects with fuller, more abstract attributes than their mere physical properties and they become similes and metaphors that attempt to connect areas of our maps of reality where the territory is more unknown.

We considered the nature and function of symbols in relation to our reality, noting that symbols create their own meaning and contexts and we have discussed how photos, like dreams are a rich source of symbolic (and object) data. We have seen that a client's photograph, as a fixed entity, allows the client and therapist to explore these meanings together. From this process, the meaning of the client's personal symbol system (as represented in the photographs) emerges, providing fuller insight and understanding. Finally, we have noted that in addition to being a rich source of symbolic data, photos serve as objective evidence of the client's history and relationship to the family and the environment. This provides a strong data base from which to proceed in therapy.

REFERENCES

Akeret, R.V. *Photoanalysis.* New York: Peter H. Wyden, Inc., 1973.

Arnheim, R. *Visual thinking.* Berkeley: University of California Press, 1971.

Bateson, G. *Steps to an ecology of mind.* New York: Ballantine Books, 1972.

Becker, E. *The birth and death of meaning.* New York: Macmillan Co., 1971.

Campbell, J. *Myths to live by.* New York: Viking Press, 1972.

Combs, A., Richards, A., & Richards, C. *Perceptual psychology.* New York: Harper and Row, 1976.

Downing, J.J., & Marmerstein, R. *Dreams and nightmares: A book of gestalt therapy sessions.* New York: Harper and Row, 1973.

Freud, S. New introductory lectures on psychoanalysis. In J. Straphey (Ed.), *Part II: Dreams.* London: The Hogarth Press, 1963.

Freud, S. *The basic writings of Sigmund Freud: The interpretation of dreams.* New York: Random House, 1938.

Grinder, J., & Bandler, R. *The structure of magic* (Vols. I & II). Palo Alto: Science and Behavior Books, 1975.

Hall, E. *The silent language.* Garden City: Anchor Press/Doubleday, 1959.

Jung, C. *The practice of psychotherapy.* New York: Pantheon, 1954.

May, R. Creativity and encounter. *American Journal of Psychoanalysis,* 1964, *24,* (1), 39-45.

Moreno, J.L. *Psychodrama* (Vol. I). Beacon, New York: Beacon House, 1972.

Naumberg, M. *Dynamically oriented art therapy: Its principles and practice.* New York: Grune and Stratton, 1966.

Ornstein, R. *The psychology of consciousness.* New York: Penguin Books, 1972.

Perls, F., Hefferline, R.F., & Goodman, P. *Gestalt therapy.* New York: Dell Publishing. 1951.

Read, H. *Icon and idea.* New York: Schocken Books, 1965.

Reusch, J. *Nonverbal communication.* Berkeley: University of California Press, 1969.

Segall, M.H., Campbell, D.T. & Herskovitz, M.J. *The influence of culture on visual perception.* Indianapolis: Bobbs-Merrill, 1966.

Woldt, A. Personal communication. Kent, Ohio: Kent State University, 1979.

Zakia, R. *Perception and photography.* Englewood Cliffs, New Jersey: Prentice-Hall, 1975.

Zinker, J. Dream work as theatre: An innovation in gestalt therapy. *Voices,* 1971, *7*(2), 17-25.

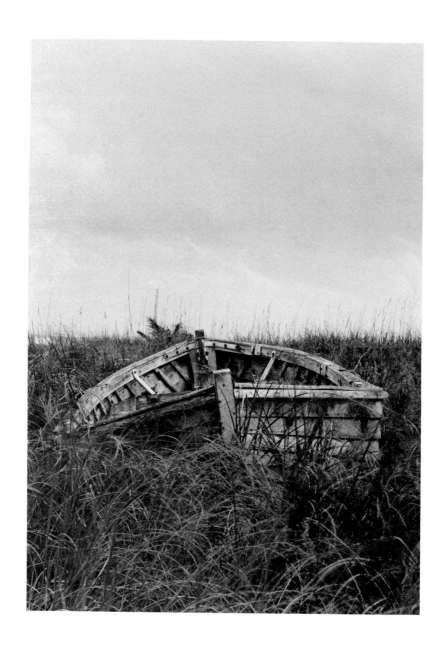

Photo by David A. Krauss

Chapter 4

The Visual Metaphor: Some Underlying Assumptions of Phototherapy

DAVID A. KRAUSS

Time it was,
And what a time it was,
It was. . .
A time of innocence,
A time of confidences.
Long ago. . .it must be. . .
I have a photograph.
Preserve your memories;
They're all that's left you.

P ILED in shoe boxes on closet shelves, pasted on bedroom mirrors, neatly arranged on the piano, or in albums, personal photographs document our experience of being alive in the world. They are graphic symbols, representations of the people, places and things in a life. They are artifacts of our existence forever framed and frozen on film. Although these portrayed images are of a past, we always respond to them in the present. The information which personal images contain affects us in many ways, defining and directing our memories of the past, and causing us to remember events from the photograph's point of view. Invariably, this influences our awareness and understanding in the here and now.

This seems to be true not only for our personal or private photographs but for public images as well.

History and behavior are not often thought to be based on mere visual images. However, there is some agreement that the ways we perceive, even the way we remember circumstances may be molded by photographs. People scarcely saw the slums until Jacob Riis photographed them. The depression sticks in memory as Walker

Evans depicted it.[1]

As part of the psychotherapeutic process, photographs, especially those of the "snapshot" variety have been used with individuals, families and groups for gathering information about the past, developing insight in the present, and offering hope and direction for a future.

Client photographs are artifacts that symbolically show relationships, contexts and the dynamics of peoples' lives. As the client responds and reflects upon these artifacts, he or she reexperiences the historical feelings associated with the images. Subsequently, the client is forced to reinterpret this information in the present. This helps clients develop skills in perceiving, feeling, thinking, behaving, and communicating.

A good deal of the power of the phototherapeutic technique derives from the photographs ability to function simultaneously as both an object, such as a picture of a family, and as a metphoric representation, such as a symbol of all families, and/or what I am reminded of when I see a family photograph. Photographs have content that is both pictorial and emotional.

In the field of psychology, an understanding of the nature of metaphor has been used for years in the areas of dream analysis, hypnosis, projective work, fantasy and art therapy. The purpose of this chapter is to focus on metaphor, its pictorial nature and how the use of photographs and visually referent language are potent therapeutic techniques. [2]It seeks to show the underlying assumptions, and to illustrate the ways in which metaphor affects us so profoundly. It seeks to answer the question, "Why phototherapy?"

CONTACTING AND COMPREHENDING THE WORLD

On a most fundamental physiological level, making correct adaptive responses to the world determines our survival. The information to make these responses derives from our auditory, kinesthetic, olfactory, gustatory and visual senses. These senses are the means by which we discover initially what is real, i.e. what will give us warmth, shelter and nourishment, and what is not real. As we mature, as we become aware and conceptualizing beings in the world, we learn to use our senses in more sophisticated ways as a means for

---

[1]Goldberg, V. Four who suggest photography has the power to shape thought. *American Photographer (7)6,* Dec. 1981, 34-38.

[2]Although not dealt with per se in this chapter, the use of the visual sense to create pictures or scenarios in our mind's eye is called imaging. The creation of visual images for developing change strategies has a long history in which this process has been used for developing personal power, inner strength or peace, changing behavior, combating disease and pain, etc. In the helping professions imaging is used in such areas as biofeedback, meditation, stress reduction, hypnosis, disease and pain control, etc. These areas have been written about fairly extensively. The book *Seeing With The Mind's Eye* by Samuels is such a good general introduction to this area. In the past few years much interesting work has been done in our culture with guided imagery in combating pain and disease. Books such as *Free Yourself From Pain* by Bresler and Turbo, *Healings from Within,* Jaffe, and *Getting Well Again* by Simonton, Matthews-Simonton, and Creighton document the potential power in these visually oriented techniques which can be used by mental health practitioners. The International Imagery Association publishes a *Journal of Mental Imagery* and it is recommended reading for those who wish to more broadly explore this area.

gathering information. In processes analogous to what Piaget has described developmentally as "accommodation and assimilation" we find that our understanding of the world derives from our ability to create anew at each level of our cognitive development, a figure and a ground, to experience differentiation, to discover ourselves as individuals in the world.

We may also consider this developmental process as the two broad categories of physical and spiritual needs in Maslow's self-actualization hierarchy. Initially our senses help us obtain physiological needs and ultimately they help us set the stage for transcendent experience. They are the materials by which we build cognition and derive our sense of wonder about the world.

Because our senses are our primary link with our reality, it follows that the more we can utilize any and/or all of our sensory inputs at any given time (up to the point of sensory overload) the more we will be in contact with the world, the more information we will have to work with as we organize responses, and the more functional and adaptive these responses can be. We seek the ability to fluidly utilize any one or combination of senses in translating that sensory input into information and action.

Authors such as Bateson and Bandler and Grinder have demonstrated that although people can and do employ all their senses to some degree, we all have favorite, sense-derived orientations for accessing or receiving and ordering incoming stimuli and for representing our reality. As basic as the process is, the dominance of a primary sensory orientation has built-in problems.

First, since the engagement of any sensory mode entails a disregarding of information from other sensory channels, some of our ability to functionally employ all of our senses may greatly diminish over time rigidifying our reality and limiting our experience.

Second, just as the language we speak influences our thought processes, each sense allows us to know things in ways specific to the sense employed. Additionally all human senses have finite limits in terms of sensitivity which prevent us from gathering fuller and more complete information from the environment. For example, we do not see the same part of the spectrum visible to bees, hear as well as canines or have olfactory abilities equal to many animals.

As we search for the real and true nature of our existence, our senses become inadequate. One might describe the problem we encounter in this search by stating somewhat paradoxically that the human situation is one in which we have enough awareness and understanding to know that there is much about our existence that we cannot be aware of or understand. Our quest for knowledge might be likened to an attempt to open an infinite number of Chinese puzzle boxes. Inside each box we open, we find another small box.

The creation of culture is a collective attempt to grapple with and solve this puzzle; it is a way of creating an aggregate of shared sensory derived perceptions and beliefs about the world in the hope that the ensuing gestalt will better approximate the truth than the average individual is able to do. The creation of culture attempts to answer for its time, and in its way, the question "What is true?" and it provides reference points from which to continue the search. Additionally, it attempts to ease individual anxiety concerning the best way to live a life by the creation of a mutually shared myth system which is sometimes called a "map of reality."

It is within the parameters of the cultural definition of reality that we compare and refine our personal versions to it. We look to the culture to create a more encompassing, "truer" map of reality than we are able to conceive of as individuals. We look to this map to supplement our own and to show us the missing territories. It becomes the scale by which we measure our experience, a way to extend our understanding. This belief is exemplified by the analogy in which a large group of individuals each with lanterns, trying to bring truth to light, gather together on a dark night. They gather together so that their combined light will illuminate more brightly and further in all directions than any one individual with his or her lantern could accomplish, thus increasing the likelihood of finding what they seek. (The underlying assumption being that the night is not infinitely dark.)

Three of the most powerful forces a culture develops to this end are religion, art, and science. They create a complex lens through which reality is viewed. While other older or more "primitive" cultures traditionally tend to view these forces in a more integrated way, contemporary western culture generally views them separately. This fragmentation of view and the disintegration of a single cultural perspective has diminished traditional certainties of belief without furnishing any one viable convincing alternative. Additionally, the constant, accelerated change and the explosion of information and knowledge which is so characteristic of this time has broadened these schisms.

Because our culture lenses no longer focus on the same things, because they have lost their powers of resolution, individuals are left more to their own devices for creating viable symbol systems on which to base their beliefs and behaviors. This is an awesome burden.

SYMBOLS AND MAP MAKING

The creation of symbols is an ongoing spontaneous activity which takes place both in and out of our awareness, while we are awake and while we dream in sleep. We constantly seek to understand the world, to cause it and our existence in it to make sense to us. We seek to create larger and more connected meaning with objects and ideas. We attempt to go beyond our logic to arrive at a more whole and deeper understanding. In paying attention to our process of symbol making we become aware of how the vast majority of these symbols are predominantly pictorial in nature.

There are many kinds of symbols cultural and personal, public and private, and there are many levels and uses of these symbols. For example, spoken language is a consciously agreed-upon symbol system, a way of giving noises created by our vocal chords generally agreed upon meanings. The earlier descriptions in this chapter of culture as a lens through which we view the world, or our creation of maps of reality, are metaphors, the figurative language derived from symbols which creates juxtapositions and new perspectives, allowing us to consider these areas of human concern in new relationships. Metaphors are information presented in ways which go beyond analytical or linear points of view, offering us the potential vehicle to expand our perspectives and to see things in a different light. (This making of metaphor is a tremendous source of power and vitality in arts, sciences, and religions.)

The spontaneous making of symbols in both the awake and the sleeping states has been the domain of concern of psychotherapy from its inception. In the early days of psychoanalysis, Freud and Jung spent much time studying their patients' symbols from accounts of their dreams and their free associations while in therapy.

There evolved the understanding that the patients' personal symbols were potent metaphors for their concerns and their present states of being. Freud further noted that visual symbols are a much truer (more useful) account of a person's concerns and processes than were verbal reports because our constant familiarity with words and their conscious combinations in sentences are more knowable and more highly defended (filtered) then our more "primitive" visual processes.

Jung was further able to demonstrate in *Man and His Symbols* (1964) the universal nature of the symbol making process and the surprisingly similar symbols that humans throughout history have used to respond to the unknown to make it comprehensible.[3] In this way the early psychoanalysists were able to glimpse into the murky workings of our unconscious processes and view what was revealed by our symbols.

Our photographs are personal symbols that have the energy to summon and demonstrate the dynamic power of our lives. They are amenable to exploration. As symbols photographs have a number of characteristics; in snapshots, for instance, the photograph serves as an artifact, icon, or totem that allows us to reconnect, with a past event in the present. Photographs are slices of the past, frozen dreams full of the dreamer's symbolism. Their form and content are determined by the photographer. Photographs also allow us to examine events and relationships in time. They therefore can be viewed as projectives, self-portraits, and/or metaphors revealing a way a photographer sees the world. They are simultaneously *of* something (dad's birthday party) and *about* something (what the data in the photograph implies regarding my relationship

---

[3]These similarities in symbol making appear to derive from the very evolution of human consciousness and the bilateral nature of the cerebral cortex. Brain research to date has shown that visual images seem to access a different part of the brain than words or writing. Visual images seem to access the nonsequential, nonlinear, more intuitive and integrative part of the brain. This been labeled by researchers as "right-brain mode" since it takes place predominantly in the right hemisphere of our brain in 97 percent of the population.

with dad, or what could be elicited about that relationship through conversation, etc.) They are symbols that we have created in the past and revitalize in the present.

From a more concrete perspective photographs are two-dimensional graphic representations of three-dimensional events that have occurred in time, arrived at by use of camera and film. They show us what an event looked like at a certain moment, from a certain angle and distance, at a certain lens opening and shutter speed, using a certain camera and film. This film is then printed in a certain way to create a graphic, symbolic representation of the event. As tenuous as the process would appear, many photographers have made images that, according to consensual validation, are good samples or good fits with reality.

Photographs allow us to remember forgotten details of our personal past and permit us to discover new truths of our universe. They show what we wore at our fifth birthday party, and what the moons of Saturn look like. They document our growing up and they permit us to glimpse inside a working human heart.

On encountering a photograph, we orient it to us by making a number of decisions and assumptions about it such as: which side is the top, what constitutes the figure in the image, what is familiar and what is unfamiliar, what is the content and how do we choose to respond to it.

When we view a personal photograph we say that the people represented in the image "are our family." As we focus on the content of the photographic image we project a "depth of field," which allows us to "know" that the house is in the background and the people are in the foreground. Without the training and benefit of being able to use the renaissance perspective we would most likely have a difficult time making the image make sense. This often happens in cultures without the benefit of renaissance perspective and for most people when they view abstract images, images from novel perspectives, and extreme close-ups or macro-photographs.

In this process we must first choose to pay more attention to the photograph than to other stimuli impinging on our senses, i.e. there is some filtering and selecting of sensory input which causes a photograph (figure) to emerge from the rest of the perceivable environment (a ground). This process is repeated and refined as we select a figure and a ground in the photograph itself. From a physiological point of view, it is interesting that the white border of most photographs is seldom perceived as figure or ground, since the strong figure-ground relationship between the border and the rest of the photograph is its most obvious aspect.

What has happened, however, is that we as viewers through our experience, needs and expectations have learned to selectively disregard certain aspects of the object and change others so that the photograph can make sense to fit into the frame of a personal cognitive map of reality, a process not unsimilar to responding to a Rorschach inkblot. As always, our past experience, present needs and expectations greatly color our ability to see in the here and now.[4]

Historically, a number of photographers have discussed the explicit metaphoric qualities of photographs and have consciously created metaphoric images in their work: Alfred Stieglitz, Ralph Hattersley, Minor White, among them. Stieglitz titled some of his images "equivalants," and attempted, for example, to symbolize metaphorically in the photograph the emotional state the photographer experienced while making the photograph. He hoped that that viewer would be able to experience, in some way, the emotions, perceptions, and/or understandings which correlate with the photographer's experience when the image was made. These photographers and others like them have operationalized sophisticated concepts of the medium and its emotive and evocative power.

John Szarkowski demonstrated in assembling the 1979 Museum of Modern Art photography exhibition, and subsequent book, *Mirrors and Windows,* that photographs are not only windows to the world which allow us to, for example, "see" our family in the picture, they are also mirrors which we project upon and have reflected back to us various aspects of our awareness. The exhibition was another in a long series of explicit affirmations of the projective and metaphorical quality of the pictorial information.

This dual quality is useful in therapy. Client photographs are not only windows that show us the "who, what, where and when" of their lives, they are also the mirrors, the symbols and the metaphors of their lives. Photographs made in the past as well as those made with instant materials during a therapy session have this quality and can be considered in this light. The client's choice of these personal symbols in the photographs and the therapeutic interpretation can bring to awareness that which formerly took place primarily at an unconscious level. Picasso has been widely quoted as saying that art is a lie which leads us closer to the truth. The same processes are involved in understanding client photographs: their literal and symbolic statements are vehicles which when explored, can also lead us closer to the truth.

THERAPEUTIC APPLICATIONS OF
THE VISUAL MODE AND METAPHOR

The therapeutic process is a process of change. It is a refocusing of feelings, thoughts, and behaviors, which help create a different outlook and greater insight. Much of this process is educational where we collaborate with clients to help them "to be" different. Since people learn in various ways, depending on

---

[4]Because viewing photographs does involve various elements of projection, all mental health practitioners have a professional obligation to be as aware and clear as possible about their personal projections, and their needs and expectations concerning client photographs. Therapists need to do their own work in this area; they need to explore their own photographs from this perspective.

motivation, readiness, amount and kind of prior learning, and the way they access, organize, and represent information, it behooves us as therapists to have
in our repertoire flexible and adaptive behavior. By engaging and understanding the visual mode and its metaphoric implications, the therapist can tap into
powerful information and communication areas creating change strategies that
will affect clients both implicitly and explicitly, as well as literally and symbolically.

As we have noted, the visual sense is dominant in our culture, and we find
that many clients also use it as their primary sensory orientation to the world.
Problems often arise for therapists with these clients in therapy when they are
asked to respond around feelings, i.e. "How do you feel about that?" These
clients' feelings are not immediately available to them because they are accessing and representating their experiences from their visual sensory orientation.
They have initial difficulty finding their feelings because they are seeing an image and can't "see" what the therapist means in terms of feelings (the kinesthetic
sense). Clinicians trained only in talking about feelings (kinesthetic and
auditory senses) may fail to make contact or much therapeutic change with
these clients.[5] As a result of this miscommunication, clients may be labeled as
"not good candidates for therapy," "resistive to therapy," or "not insightful" (!).
These clients can, of course, be in touch with their feelings, but these feelings
must be reached through the visual orientation, i.e. "When you don't see your
way out of this situation, how does your world look and how does that make
you feel?" What is important to understand here is the use of visually referent
language as a way to make contact and be in communication with the client.
Therapists should consciously use a vocabulary based on visually referent
words and phrases such as I have used throughout this chapter. They include,
for example: *change in outook, viewpoint,* or *point of view, get the picture, flash of insight, sharper focus, greater depth of field, bring to light, occluded perception, blind spot,
greater acuity, different angle, vignetted details, near sighted, far sighted, myopic, look away
from, distorted self-image,* etc.

In working with clients, their initial willingness to bring in and discuss
photos can be a metaphoric indication of their trust level and readiness to be involved in the therapeutic process. Clients who bring in one or two selected images may be symbolically making quite different statements than those who
bring in the album or those who dump a couple of shoe boxes full of snapshots
on the desk. Also, the number of different kinds of photos clients bring into the
session gives the therapist much information about the depth and diversity of
their world and the range of subjects that can be viewed and discussed, i.e. a
metaphor for norms and rules about being and experiencing are presented.

Additionally, on the same metaphoric level working with client photographs

---

[5]The recent article by W. Falzett in the *Journal of Counseling Psychology* 28(4) presents some experimental
results confirming that subjects perceived counselors more trustworthy when the counselors used predicates
that matched the subjects' primary representational system.

brings the client's process to light. For example, is the client shy or resistive in presenting photographs? What is said about the images and how is she or he organizing the presentation? The therapist sees how clients organize and present photos and how they interact in a relatively unthreatening therapeutic encounter. The therapist also learns how clients define themselves and the amount of ease and/or degree of difficulty the client has in organizing, presenting, and changing subject matter, angle, and point of view. Combined with the photographs themselves this information gives the therapist quick and efficient access to a client's history and present strengths and weaknesses, creating a baseline from which to measure change. By engaging in the use of the phototherapeutic techniques, the therapist develops a relatively comprehensive picture of the client's way of being in the world which is in sharper focus and has greater depth of field.

Even more fundamentally, the profound power of photographic images to function metaphorically as catalysts to insight and understanding can be demonstrated from the following two short examples where personal photographs were allowed to speak for themselves. I had the opportunity to work with a divorced woman who was willing to look at her family photos. What we saw in the images made by her husband was that he had a hard time facing and making visual contact with her. He would only photograph her obliquely or "on a pedestal" where she was somehow above him. He also would not photograph her at close range, preferring some distance. This behavior changed when he photographed their young child. He would make images at a much closer range, often eliminating the mother's head or other parts of her body but always including the child. Reviewing these images for her was an experience of understanding in a new way some of the problems and dynamics of the relationship that had been there pictorially since courtship. Her ability to see this information in the photographs allowed her to feel better and to resolve emotionally some things she knew intellectually. Discussing these photos was an affirmation for her.

Another woman who was a therapist herself asked me to go over her photos so that she could see first hand how photography might be used with clients. She had a fairly large number of snapshots and I asked her to select a few that were the most important to her. She proceeded to choose about fifteen or twenty. I spread them out on the table before us and started asking questions about the images while I looked for themes. Two images caught my attention. One was of her mother and herself at the kitchen table in mother's house. Mother was seated and P. was behind her mother in a position where she had her arm around mother's shoulder and her head next to mothers's breast — a look that she later described as "loving, nurturing, and taking care of." In a second photograph she assumed what appeared to me to be a similar posture on a living room chair with a (now former) lover. When I moved the other photographs aside and presented these two to her side by side, she put her palm to her forehead and had what we refer to in therapy as an aha! experience. She said that a number of things suddenly made sense to her and proceeded to elaborate on this experience. In this case the metaphor created by presentation of the two images side by side was enough to create a powerful discovery for this woman around her personal issues of independence, nurturance and dependence. These two cases illustrate two ways in which we commonly use the visual metaphor in therapy: to show some new reality visually by the discussion and positioning of photos, and to make clear the concerns or themes to which a client is at least partially blind.

This chapter has looked at the visual: the visual sense as it accesses and represents information, visually referent language, and the various ways photographic images may function as symbols and metaphor. It has attempted to demonstrate the potency and primacy of the visual in our search for understanding the world and our successful survival, and how the power inherent in visuals can be utilized in therapy. By actively working with all appropriate aspects of the visual metaphor and encouraging clients to explore the boundaries of their vision, and to gain insight, the clients and their picture of the world changes. The evolved perception and vision enlarges the clients' ability to view the world and to create their place in it.

REFERENCES

Arnheim, R., *Visual thinking*. Berkley: University of California Press, 1971.

Bandler, R., & Grinder, J., *Structure of magic I*. Palo Alto: Science and Behavior Books, 1975.

Bateson, G. *Steps to an ecology of mind*. New York: Ballantine Books, 1972.

Freud, S., *The basic writings of Sigmund Freud*. New York: Random House, 1938.

Hattersley, R., *Discover yourself through photography*. New York: Morgan and Morgan, 1971.

Jung, C., *Man and his symbols*. Garden City, New York: Doubleday, 1964.

Read, H., *Icon and idea*. New York: Schocken Books, 1965.

Segall, M., Campbell, D., & Herskovitz, M., *The influence of culture on visual perception*. Indianapolis: Bobbs-Merrill, 1966.

Stieglitz, A., *The Aperture history of photography series, Book 3*. Millerton, New York: Aperture, 1976.

Szarkowski, J., *Mirrors and windows*. Boston: New York Graphic Society, 1979.

White, M. Equivalance: the perennial trend. In N. Lyons (ed.), *Photographers on photography*. Englewood Cliffs, New Jersey: Prentice-Hall, 1966.

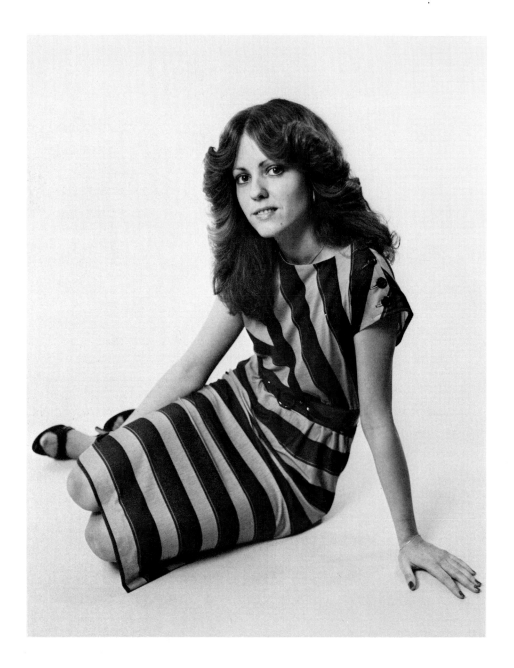

Photo by David G. Hall

Chapter 5

Photographic
Self-Confrontation
as Therapy

JERRY L. FRYREAR

CONFRONTATION, SELF-CONCEPT AND SELF-ESTEEM

CONFRONTATION is a term and concept encountered frequently in the psychotherapy literature. The therapist is said to confront the client when he or she points out contradictions among the client's verbal statements, between verbal and nonverbal communications, or between actions and statements about those actions. The therapist may confront the client's behavior and fantasies, forcing him or her to compare the behavior and fantasies with real or probable consequences of actions. The assumption is that the client can not or will not confront himself or herself, and that the confrontation will lead to insight and a desire to change on the part of the client.

Often, statements, nonverbal communications, fantasies and actions are about or related to the client's self-concept and self-esteem. A client may say, "I hate myself," "My legs are too skinny," "I wish I were prettier," "I can't forgive myself." The client may make a wry face when discussing his appearance. A client may have day dreams or night dreams that revolve around themes of self-identity and self-esteem. A client may try to disfigure or destroy herself or himself.

We have concepts of ourselves as possessing certain identities and belonging to certain groups or categories. Indeed, it is misleading to refer to one's self-concept as a unidimensional construct. More accurately, we conceptualize ourselves as belonging to a great many categories. For example, I conceive of myself as a *person*, belonging to the species *Homo sapiens*. I also place myself in the categories of U.S. citizen, man, professor, writer, father, husband, son, brother, psychologist, taxpayer and person with brown hair, to name a few. I

All of the photographs reproduced in this chapter are of models rather than actual clients because of laws prohibiting the publications of photographs of juveniles. However, the models portray poses that are like those of the clients.

71

have many self-concepts, not *a* self-concept. These self-concepts are possible because I am aware of my self as an object, can perceive certain physical and behavioral attributes of myself, and can conceptualize those attributes by comparing them with other people's, and with information I have learned.

There seems to be a great deal of confusion between the terms *self-concept* and *self-esteem*. Self-concept, as I have said, is a category that we place ourselves into, such as "husband." That particular concept depends on the awareness of oneself as an organism in a specific relationship to another, namely marriage. There are other relationship self-concepts of course, including "father" and "son." Furthermore, these three examples of "husband," "father" and "son" all have to do with family relationships, involving genetic and marital bonds. For the sake of convenience, we could group all such family self-concepts together and speak of one's family self-concept as if it were a single construct. Likewise, we could group all other relationship self-concepts into a nonfamilial grouping and call that construct "social self-concept." Such a construct would include self-concepts of "friend," "colleague," "companion," and so forth. Taking this discussion further, we could identify other groups of self-concepts such as "religious self-concept," "physical self-concept," "socioeconomic self-concept," "culture self-concept," and "vocational self-concept." All such groupings are somewhat arbitrary, and are made for convenience.

Some groupings, or constructs, of self-concepts are psychologically more meaningful than others. Generally speaking, the more psychologically meaningful constructs are the ones that we esteem. That is, we tend to evaluate self-concepts along a positive-negative dimension. It is possible to think of a person as having hundreds of self-concepts, with each one evaluated, or esteemed, as having a certain amount of worth. More conveniently, we think of a person as having a limited number of self-concept constructs, each with its accompanying self-worth. The self-concept constructs that tend to be evaluated by one's self are ones that depend on our physical condition or our actions, rather than on some other attributes such as our blood type, which is not under our direct control. So family selves, social selves, physical selves, religious selves and vocational selves tend to be more important psychologically than some other constructs. Self-esteem, then, is the evaluation of worth that we give to a self-concept. A grouping of these evaluations, incorporating some psychologically meaningful category or contruct such as "family self," then becomes a self-esteem construct.

There have been several attempts to identify and measure psychologically meaningful self-concept and self-esteem constructs. One of the most successful is that of William Fitts, who developed the Tennessee Self-Concept Scale (TSCS). The TSCS contains five major groupings of self-concepts, named "physical," "moral-ethical," "social," "family," and "personal." The scale contains items within each of the constructs that reflect more specific self-concepts, and each item is rated, by the person filling out the scale, along an evaluative dimension. Thus, each of the five constructs of self-concept leads to scores for self-esteem. Finally, the five constructs of self-esteem are summed to derive an overall level of self-esteem that can be compared with normative samples of other people who have taken the scale. Unfortunately, Fitts adds to the semantic confusion by calling this overall measure a self-concept score rather than a self-esteem score. (See Fitts et al., 1969-1972, for a detailed discussion of self-concept and the TSCS scales.)

Self-confrontation as a therapeutic concept rests on the notion of self-concept and self-esteem and the corresponding theoretical stance of a divided self — the self as an object to be perceived, classified, and evaluated, and the self as an observer, to perceive, classify and evaluate. The observing self continually perceives attributes of the objective self, classifies (conceptualizes) and evaluates (esteems) the concepts in an ongoing process. The esteem, or worth, that the observing self places on the observed self is largely a result of the esteem, or worth, that significant others have placed on those constructs during the person's lifetime (see Rogers, 1959). Self-confrontation requires a third perspective, in addition to the observing self and the objective self, that of *observing the observer*. That third perspective is difficult for people to achieve, without help from someone else. Or perhaps I should say that the third perspective, as a therapeutically critical one, is difficult for people to achieve. People do observe the self-process in themselves but in an unquestioning way.

Therapeutic confrontation begins initially with a therapist. The therapist acts as an observer of the self-process, commenting on the perceptual, conceptual and evaluative dimensions. Usually, the confrontation is centered on the evaluative part of the process, because that part is most vulnerable to individual interpretations. In some unusual cases, it is possible that a client will perceive attributes of himself or herself that are almost certainly not true (such as a foul odor, extra limbs, or a rotting stomach) or will classify attributes in ways that are not consensually validated (such as assignment of oneself to the category of "demon" or some famous historical personage). By confronting the self-process, the therapist hopes that the client will change the ways in which he/she perceives, classifies or evaluates the various attributes of self. Finally, the therapist encourages the client to take over that monitoring job. That is, the therapist moves from confrontation toward self-confrontation, with those clients in which distortions of self-concept or self-esteem are an important or central part of the psychopathology. It should be noted that self-concept or self-esteem are not central to all problems for which people are referred to therapists. The therapist must judge whether self-confrontation is an appropriate goal/technique for each case.

When self-esteem of one or more self-concepts is low, therapeutic self-confrontation may be indicated. It is not uncommon for prospective clients to have generally low self-esteem with respect to one or more concepts of themselves. The traditional neurotic categories of conversion reactions, obsessions and compulsions, and depressive reactions are especially likely to correlate with low self-esteem. Also, juvenile deliquency is thought by many theorists to be the direct result of low self-esteem. Delinquent youth are trying, in a maladaptive way, to make up for what they perceive as physical, social, or other deficits in themselves. They may not be deficient by other people's standards, but they believe they are and that belief motivates their behavior.

PHOTOGRAPHIC SELF-CONFRONTATION

Photographic self-confrontation involves providing the client with visual information about the self as an object. The information can be in the form of still photos, film, videotape playback, or even mirrors. The rationale is that this visual information about the self will correct misperceptions, force reconceptualizations, or enhance the esteem in which the observing self holds the objective self. Social, family, physical, and other attributes can be captured on film or tape and used in confrontive ways. Whether the self-confrontation is therapeutic depends on the selection of the client, the selection of attributes to confront, and the methods of confrontation used. Self-confrontation is not automatically or necessarily therapeutic. Regardless of the specific technique, the provision of a visual display of one's self demands that one observe one's self, and virtually forces the third perspective of observing the self-process. Danet (1968), speaking of video replay, states that now patients can not only see themselves as others see them but can react to their own behavior in a way similar to that of the others with whom they have interacted. Their reactions to themselves provide them with still more information.

Family phototherapists may rely on historical photographs from the client's family album for confrontational purposes. That method is discussed by Alan Entin in Chapter 7. It is rich in diagnostic information relative to the client's family self-concepts and the dynamics of the family system. By using historical photographs from the family, the family album method also allows the client to observe the family self-concept and self-esteem process over the life span, possibly several years, in the supportive atmosphere of the therapy room.

Other family phototherapists prefer to photograph or videotape the family as the members interact in the therapy session. That visual information provides the client with elaborate data related to his or her family self-concept and self-esteem, relative to the other family members. For example, a client may notice that he always looks down when father speaks to him, an indication of lowered self-esteem when in the father's presense. That data may contradict the client's statements or even beliefs about his relationship to the father, and lead to a more honest assessment of the family self-esteem and then to strategies for enhancing that self-esteem.

Other phototherapists who have less of an orientation toward family therapy and more of an orientation toward the individual are likely to use visual methods directly in the therapy sessions with individual clients or groups of clients. In the remainder of this chapter I shall describe several efforts to use therapeutic photographic self-confrontation of physical and social attributes in an effort to enhance self-esteem and improve behaviors in those areas.

PHYSICAL SELF-CONFRONTATION

There are several reasons why physical self-confrontation is or can be therapeutic. One possibility is that a client simply does not know what he or she looks like, and the visual self-confrontation provides the client with previously unknown information. So, for example, a teenager may think of himself as ugly or otherwise visually unique in the absence of "objective" evidence to the contrary. His opinion of his appearance may be due to real or imagined feedback from other people, who may be biased and hostile toward him. The photographic self-portrait then gives the client an additional bit of evidence that, when compared with other photographs or other opinions, may change his perception of himself, convince him that his opinion was erroneous, and thus enhance self-esteem. Logic and empirical evidence supports this view.

Logically, there is no reason why people would have an image of themselves that corresponds to other people's. We see ourselves in mirrors, which provides a reversed and reduced image; we see ourselves in stiffly posed photographs, also greatly reduced in size; we rarely see ourselves from the rear or even from the side — other people see us from these angles frequently.

Empirically, there is evidence that there is in fact a range of self-recognition abilities among people. Some of us are much better at recognizing visual displays of ourselves than others. Self-recognition deficits, compared with "normal" ability, have been documented by Cornelison and Arsenian (1960), Pollack, Karp, Kahn and Goldfarb (1962) and Fryrear, Kodera and Kennedy (1981). Tom Kodera, Martha Kennedy, and I have discovered three people who could not recognize photographic slides of themselves, although they could recognize slides of their friends.

If the phototherapist is assuming that photographic self-confrontation will educate the client and somehow "correct" the client's body image, it would be well to try to measure the body image as a test of the assumption. One could use an indirect measure such as the physical self-concept subscale of the Tennessee Self-Concept Scale, or a direct method such as a measure of the individual's ability to recognize photographs of himself or herself. The clarity of the photographs could be varied by changing the background lighting, varying the focus, or changing the light intensity of a slide projector (a detailed description of an optic system for measuring self-recognition can be found in an article by Fryrear, Kodera and Kennedy, 1981). In cases of low physical self-esteem, it is possible that a person has a very accurate body image and simply does not like it. It is unlikely that visual self-confrontation would be therapeutic with such a person, and in fact may be damaging.

A related therapeutic rationale is that a person knows what he or she looks like, but not what he or she *could* look like under other circumstances. A client may lack grooming skills and may never have seen herself or himself with combed hair and neat clothes. Visual feedback of a well-groomed self may be rewarding to the person and may result in higher self-esteem and enhanced appearance and hygiene.

Conversely, it is probably dangerous to show a client what he or she could look like in undesirable circumstances, such as in a drunken state. Such a confrontation method may simply provide clients with selective evidence that supports their own self-fulfilling prophecies. As Hosford (1980), writing about self-modeling notes, "(Clients) particularly observe or consciously choose to observe those suspected discrepancies between their actual and desired behavior. By focusing primarily on their perceived mistakes they not ony fail to observe and strengthen the more positive behaviors being modeled, but they learn to associate feelings of unpleasantness with the self-observation process itself" (p. 51). I would add that Hosford's analysis applies also to physical appearance. Clients may choose to attend to negatively perceived physical attributes of themselves. It does not seem wise for a therapist to accentuate that self-defeating process.

My colleagues and I have carried out five studies that involve photographic physical self-confrontation as a primary method. Three were therapeutically successful. One successful study was with male juvenile delinquents, one with fourth-grade school children, and one with disadvantaged boys in a group home.

In the first project, male juvenile delinquents with low physical self-esteem were identified with the TSCS questionnaire. The boys were divided into pairs and, over a five-week period, took pictures of each other. As the photographs were developed and returned, each boy pasted them into a self-portrait scrapbook. The poses were specified by the therapists and included various camera angles, postures, facial expressions of emotions, bodily expressions of emotions and pantomiming of everyday activities.

Session I (Head Angles)
1. Head — full front
2. Head — 3/4 right front
3. Head — 3/4 left front
4. Head — 3/4 right rear
5. Free Shot

Session III (Postures)
1. Standing
2. Sitting in chair
3. Lying prone
4. Lying supine
5. Free Shot

Session V (Facial Expressions)
1. Happy

Session II (Head Angles)
1. Head — full rear
2. Head — 3/4 left rear
3. Head — right side
4. Head — left side
5. Free Shot

Session IV (Postures)
1. Kneeling
2. Sitting on floor
3. Leaning
4. Squatting
5. Free Shot

Session VI (Facial Expressions)
1. Fearful

2. Sad

3. Angry

4. Pouting

5. Free Shot

Session VII (Body Expressions)

1. Happy

2. Sad

3. Angry

4. Pouting

5. Free Shot

Session IX (Pantomiming Activities)

1. Washing Face

2. Brushing Teeth

3. Combing Hair

4. Putting on Shoes

5. Free Shot

Session XI

Five Free Shots

2. Disgusted

3. Thoughtful

4. Surprised

5. Free Shot

Session VIII (Body Expressions)

1. Fearful

2. Disgusted

3. Thoughtful

4. Surprised

5. Free Shot

Session X (PantomimingActivities)

1. Acting Hot

2. Acting Cold

3. Buttoning Shirt

4. Buckling Belt

5. Free Shot

Session XII

Five Free Shots

By the end of the project each boy had approximately 60 pictures of himself in the scrapbook. Further questionnaire data revealed that the overall self-esteem of the boys improved over the course of the project (Fryrear, Nuell and Ridley, 1974).

In the second project, Ammerman and Fryrear (1975) extended the method into the realm of delinquency prevention. The purpose of the project was to identify children who suffered from low self-esteem and to try to enhance their self-esteem through photographic feedback before the low self-esteem could lead to a pattern of maladaptive behavior. Fourth-grade children with low self-esteem were identified through questionnaires and teachers' ratings. The children were then invited to participate in a phototherapy project similar to the first project with the delinquent boys. The children took pictures of each other, and a counselor (Ammerman) helped each child construct a self-portrait scrapbook while encouraging the children to discuss the photographs. The project was successful in diminishing classroom behaviors that have been linked to low self-esteem.

The third project (Milford, Swank and Fryrear, 1981) was an attempt to enhance institutionalized boys' self-esteem, social skills and grooming through a photography program as a means to achieve visual self-confrontation. The method was similar to the two studies cited above and was successful in improving sociability, grooming and group living behavior.

Other researchers have reported therapeutic outcomes of photographic self-confrontation. Cornelison and Arsenian (1960) showed schizophrenic patients photographs of themselves and discussed the viewing experiences with them. They reported positive changes in psychotic state in some patients, catharsis of

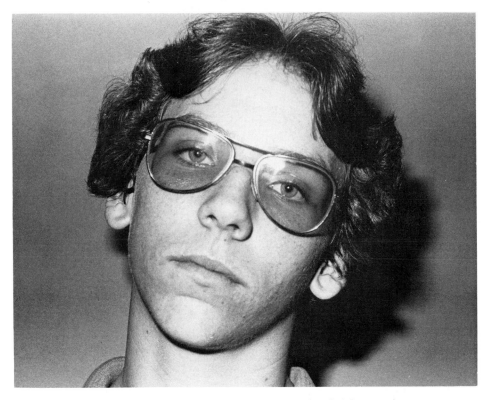

Figure 5-1. Craig attempts to portray anger using facial expressions.

some patients, and a focusing of attention upon the self. They remarked, "Since self-confrontation focuses perception upon an external image of self, this may bring a psychotic individual into better contact with the realistic self" (p. 7).

Miller (1962) used photographic self-confrontation with psychotic patients in a state hospital. He photographed the patients and displayed the photographs on their ward. Although no significant improvement in psychotic symptoms was apparent, the activity did result in increased socialization among patients and between staff and patients.

Spire (1973) used photos in a self-confrontation program with chronic schizophrenic women in a state hospital. He reported increased communication, enhanced interpersonal relations, positive behavior change, and more positive self-evaluations.

In two studies using photographic self-confrontation with delinquent girls, my colleagues and I have failed to demonstrate therapeutic effects. In one project (Fryrear and Nuell, 1973), delinquent girls were taught numerous modeling poses and were photographed modeling their own clothes. The photographs were returned to the girls and they were helped to develop self-portrait scrapbooks. We reasoned that the modeling poses were specifically designed to be flattering and that the photographs would show the girls at their

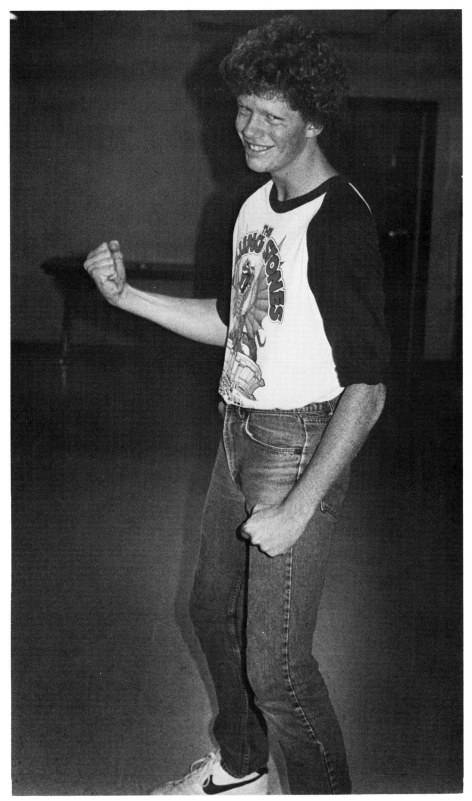

Figure 5-2. Peter attempts to portray anger using body expressions. Note the contradiction between his body and his face.

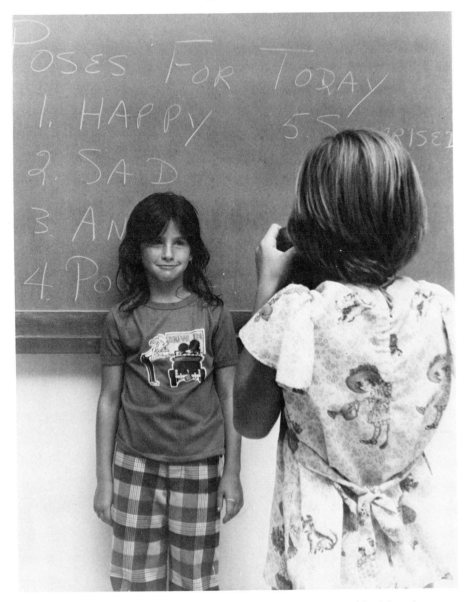

Figure 5-3. Fourth graders take part in phototherapy project conducted by Mary Ammerman and Jerry L. Fryrear.

best. Over the course of the six-week project the girls' counselors reported that the girls looked forward to the photographic sessions. Self-esteem question-naires, however, did not show positive results. The reasons are not clear but may have to do with the modeling training. The training was done by two love-ly female college students who had been part-time models, against whom the girls may have been comparing themselves. It is possible that, by comparison,

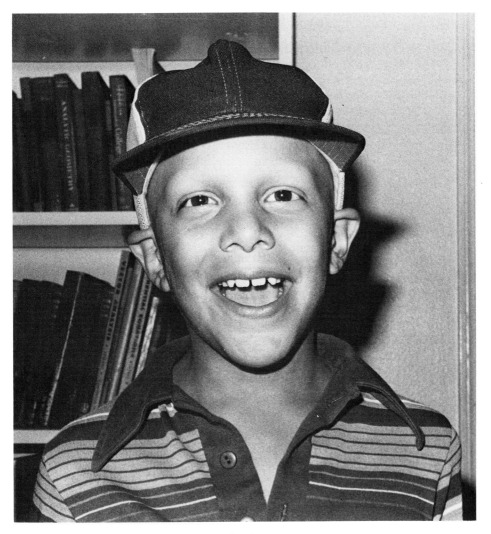

Figure 5-4. Daniel poses for full-face camera angle portrait.

the girls felt less pretty and therefore less worthy.

When we carried out the second project with delinquent girls, we did not stress appearance (Vardell, McClellan and Fryrear, 1982). Rather, we used the photography as in integral part of six, two-hour group therapy sessions. The girls introduced themselves by posing for and describing a Polaroid snapshot of themselves and, at the end of the project, by posing for and describing a farewell portrait. During the sessions the girls photographed themselves and each other from many camera angles, in mirrors, in automobiles, in unusual clothing and with various expressions. There were twelve activities in all, half of them individual assignments and half with partners. The activities and the purposes for them follow:

Activity #1

Introductory Self-Portrait (Individual)

PURPOSE: This exercise sets the tone of the program by asking the participants to use a visual mode as an introduction. It is an initial and not too threatening self-confrontation and can give the therapist some clues as to the participant's level of self-awareness and self-esteem. The exercise also aids in eliciting verbal interchange among the group members and will serve to document change when compared with later photographs.

Activity #2

Creative Hands (Partners)

PURPOSE: This second exercise is a continuation of self-presentation, this time using hands instead of face. In addition, the participants are encouraged to express themselves in a creative way, perhaps an unusual way, with the hope that they will begin to think and perceive in ways contrary to their history.

Because the participants work in pairs on this exercise, it also fosters socialization and cooperation.

Activity #3

Dog's Eye View and Bird's Eye View (Individual)

PURPOSE: This exercise is a further encouragement to creative perception. The participant must try to perceive his/her environment in ways that are new to him/her. It is hoped that these different points of view will facilitate more flexible, less stereotyped perceptions in the participants' everyday lives.

Activity #4

Creative Hair (Partners)

PURPOSE: This fourth exercise is a continuation of self-presentation — this time using hair. In addition, the participants are encouraged to express themselves in a creative way, perhaps an unusual way, with the hope that they will begin to think and perceive in ways contrary to their history. This exercise also fosters socialization and cooperation.

Activity #5

Opposites (Individual)

PURPOSE: The "opposites" exercise is designed to promote the self-actualization goal of synergy, the ability to see opposites as meaningfully related. Furthermore, it is a visual example of George Kelly's "personal constructs," allowing the participants and the therapist to examine the ways in which the participant constructs the world (Kelly, 1955). This exercise is also an exercise in creativity, and is similar to activities 2, 3 and 4.

Activity #6

Facemaking (Partners)

PURPOSE: "Facemaking" is an exercise in aligning facial expressions with inner emotions. It deals with nonverbal communication, and is especially valuable as a check on how well one communicates emotions to others. Both the photograph and the partner provide checks on the intended communications. Because the exercise uses partners, it is also designed to provide practice in recognizing particular emotions in others.

Activity #7

Pictures From Different Camera Angles (Individual)

PURPOSE: This exercise is a further encouragement to creative perception. The participant must try to perceive his/her environment in ways that are new to him/her. It is hoped that these different points of view will facilitate more flexible, less stereotyped perceptions in the participants' everyday lives.

The manner in which the participant carries out the assignment can provide the therapist with information regarding the participant's perceptions of his/her "psychological niches" (see Ailler et al., Chapter 6).

Activity #8

Mirror Mirror (Partners)

PURPOSE: This exercise provides participants an opportunity to see themselves from unusual angles and can therefore promote greater self-awareness and, perhaps, self-esteem. Because it is a partners activity, it also promotes cooperation and socialization.

Activity #9

Free Picture (Individual)

PURPOSE: By allowing freedom of choice at this point in the program, the therapist encourages responsibility and lets the participants know that they have now mastered the art and mechanics of photography to the extent necessary for such freedom. This unstructured period should contribute to enhanced self-esteem and a sense of mastery.

Activity #10

Wearing Different Clothes (Partners)

PURPOSE: To the extent that the participants wear clothing usually worn by other people, this exercise is a visual metaphor for empathy — trying to experience the world of another person. To the extent that the participants wear clothing that they normally would not, the exercise serves to help sharpen identities and broaden experiences.

Activity #11

Termination Self-Portrait (Individual)

PURPOSE: The termination self-portrait is a visual goodbye as well as an opportunity to document any change that has occurred during the program. It is also a way of symbolically prolonging the group experience through the exchange of these photographs, if the participants wish.

Activity #12

Scrapbook (Group)

PURPOSE: This final exercise allows the participants to review the program through the photographs and to arrange the photographs from the exercises in some manner that is meaningful as well as artistic. As a group exercise it promotes socialization and a sense of belonging.

A self-esteem questionnaire and behavior ratings by the staff did not show significant changes. We do not know why. It is possible that a longer program would be more effective. It is also possible that, for some unexplained reason, visual self-confrontation is not therapeutic with adolescent girls. This is an important issue and needs to be addressed by researchers. We know virtually nothing about matching potential clients with the most appropriate visual treatment modality.

SOCIAL SELF-CONFRONTATION

Because so much of social interaction involves verbal and subtle nonverbal

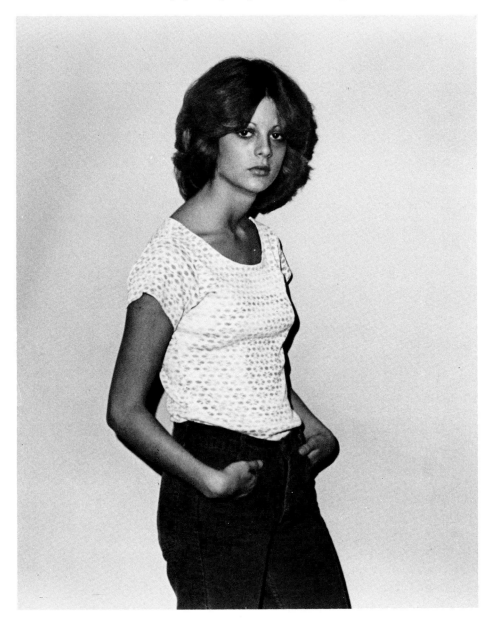

Figure 5-5. Sharon chose this pose for her introductory self-portrait.

communication patterns, most attempts at using visual self-confrontation methods for social skills training have employed video technology. Video, unlike still photography, allows replay of audio and movement. Because this book is concerned with still phototherapy, I shall not discuss videotherapy here. For information on social skills training using video self-confrontation see Berger (1978), Fryrear (1979), and Fryrear and Fleshman (1981).

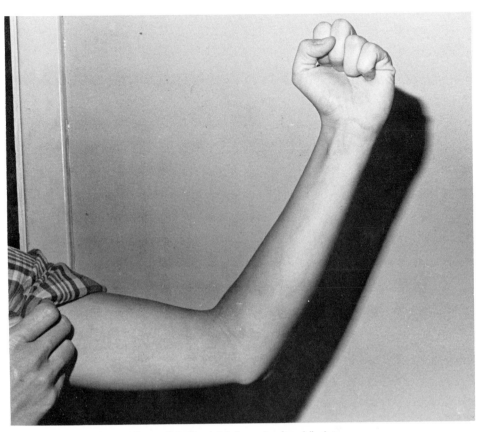

Figure 5-6. Patricia's "creative hands" picture.

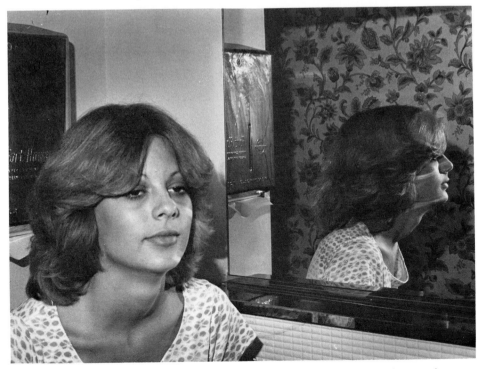

Figure 5-7. Sharon poses in front of the mirror for multiple camera angle portrait.

We have carried out one still photography study using self-confrontation of social interactions (Fryrear, Nuell and White, 1977). Using the TSCS as a screening instrument, we identified delinquent boys who had low social self-esteem. The boys were divided into trios and each boy took pictures of the other two engaging in positive social interactions — team sports, greetings, cooperative work.

As the first meeting with the subjects was primarily an acquainting and introducing experience, picture poses depicting the everyday social interaction of greeting another person were incorporated:

Greetings

    1. Regular handshake.
    2. "Power" handshake.
    3. Slapping partner amiably on the back.
    4. Being slapped on back by partner.
    5. Slapping partner on shoulder.
    6. Being slapped on shoulder.
7-12. "Free" poses: Partners greeted each other in ways initiated by each individual pair.

The boys worked in pairs for these poses; two copies of each print were made so that both members of each pair received his own copy.

The second set of poses consisted of the following:

Cooperative Activities for Two

    1. Offering a cigarette to partner.
    2. Being offered a cigarette.
    3. Lighting a cigarette for partner.
    4. Receiving a light.
    5. Dealing cards to partner.
    6. Being dealt cards.
    7. Cooperatively carrying a bench or chair.
    8. Writing on partner's back.
9-12. Free poses with same partner.

Again, two copies of each pose were printed.

For the third set of pictures, the boys posed in triads and the therapists took the snapshots. Three copies of the following were made:

Cooperative Activities for Three

    1. Being carried. Each boy took his turn being carried by the others in a cross-arm lift.

2. Triad pyramid. Each boy took his turn on top of the pyramid being supported by the other two members of his team.
3. Jumpball. Each boy took a turn throwing the ball while the others volleyed.
4. Free poses.

The fourth set of poses consisted of boxing poses with the boys again working in pairs. They were:

Boxing

1. Nose jab to partner.
2. Nose jab from partner.
3. Upper cut to partner.
4. Upper cut from partner.
5. Cross cut to partner.
6. Cross cut from partner.
7. Body jab to partner.
8. Body jab from partner.
9-12. Free boxing poses.

For the final session the following poses were used:

Grooming

1. Tying partner's tie.
2. Having tie tied by partner.
3. Shining partner's shoes.
4. Having shoes shined by partner.
5. Brushing partner's clothes.
6. Having clothes brushed by partner.
7. Cutting partner's hair (pantomimed).
8. Having hair cut by partner (pantomimed).
9-12. Free poses involving cooperative grooming activities.

As in the physical self-confrontation studies, the boys constructed scrapbooks of themselves. They documented their ability to carry out social activities adequately. The overall self-esteem of these boys improved over the course of the project.

VISUAL SELF-CONFRONTATION AS AN ADJUNCT TO VERBAL THERAPY

The studies summarized above have in common photographic self-confrontation as a therapeutic technique. The studies also included some counseling, or at least discussion, adjunctive to the visual self-confrontation.

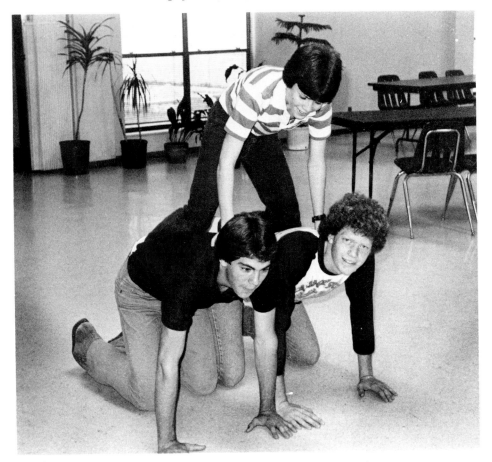

Figure 5-8. One of the exercises requiring cooperation.

The addition of the visual self-confrontation to the verbal discussion and counseling may enhance the therapeutic value of the latter because the visual self-image evokes strong arousal in the viewer which "primes" the viewer for therapeutic change. From a psychoanalytic point of view, anxiety aroused by viewing one's self in a photograph may result in heightened and more adaptive ego functions, perhaps mature ego mechanisms in place of immature or narcissistic ones. Certainly, visual or auditory self-confrontation can arouse one's anxiety (see Holzman, Rousy and Snyder, 1966). It is unlikely, however, that the increased anxiety "automatically" results in therapeutic gain. What is more likely is that the state of arousal makes the client more open to therapeutic intervention and perhaps more suggestible. Following this assumption, photographic self-confrontation would be used by therapists as affect-arousing stimuli, adjunctive to other modes of therapy.

The "arousal" rationale for visual self-confrontation as therapy has support from the theory of objective self-awareness developed by Duval and Wicklund (1972). A state of objective self-awareness occurs whenever one is confronted

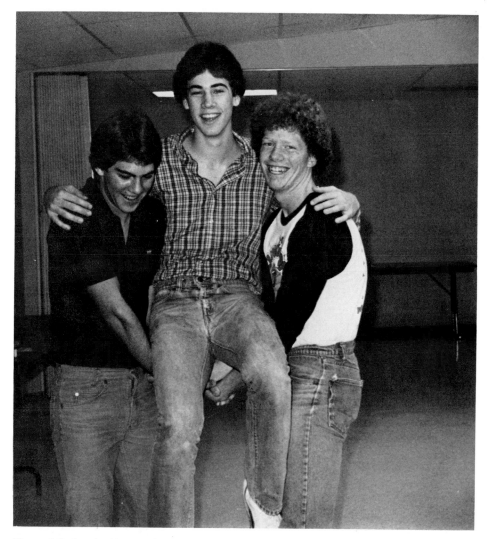

Figure 5-9. Another cooperative exercise. These exercises foster social self-esteem and cooperation.

with oneself as an object, such as when one views one's own photograph. That
state of objective self-awareness leads to a comparison of one's objective self
with an internalized standard. If the comparison is such that the viewer is
aware of a negative discrepancy between the standard and the objective self, a
state of aversive arousal exists and the person will try to escape the state of objective self-awareness. If escape is not possible, then he or she will eventually
attempt to change the objective self, changing either behavior or appearance.
Of course, the therapist would have to keep the client in a state of objective self-
awareness for a period of time necessary for change to occur. That period is no
doubt different for different people, but Wicklund (1975) has reported

behavioral changes in relatively short periods of time. In my opinion, this is a point in favor of group phototherapy. The mutually supportive atmosphere of a group would help insure that each client continues in therapy long enough to realize benefits.

Hung and Rosenthal (1981) conclude that visual feedback of videotaped self has "its maximum impact when conjoined with other therapies." Their social theory framework seems to apply to photographic feedback as well. Hung and Rosenthal point out that self-efficacy and outcome expectation, steered by personal cognitions about reality, influence the effects of visual confrontation. They emphasize that it is important to specify the meaning (message-value) of feedback. In their words, "how people are oriented to observe themselves and to discriminate message content will affect the meaning clients extract from videotaped replay" (p. 53). In other words, visual self-confrontation does not occur in a social/environmental vacuum. The phototherapist must prepare the client for the self-confrontation experience if maximum benefit (and avoidance of negative consequences) is to occur.

Hall (1983) states the case for carefully prepared visual self-confrontation succinctly. "Photographs of oneself are a potent source of feedback regarding personal appearance. Potent feedback, however, can be negative as well as positive. It seems sensible that if a therapist is to provide a client the opportunity of having photographs of himself, that it would be useful to have a degree of control over the process of generating the photographs such that the results will have the best possibility of providing positive feedback." Hall, in his phototherapy, provides "controlled self-confrontation," directing the client through the four phases of collecting information, photographing, processing of film, and viewing the photographs in such a way that the total experience is a positive, therapeutic one.

Summary

In this chapter, I have discussed the constructs of self-concept, self-esteem and self-confrontation and related those constructs to the therapeutic technique of photographic confrontation of the client. Data were presented in defense of photographic confrontation of social self and physical self. It seems likely that maximum benefit can be derived from photographic self-confrontation when the confrontation is controlled by the therapist such that the client concentrates on positive aspects of the confrontation and when the visual confrontation is part of a more comprehensive therapeutic approach, such as cognitive or phenomenological therapy.

REFERENCES

Ammerman, M.S., and Fryrear, J.L. Photographic enhancement of children's self esteem. *Psychology in the Schools.* 1975, *12*(3), 319-225.

Berger, M.M. *Videotape techniques in psychiatric training and treatment,* 2nd ed. New York: Brunner/ Mazel, 1978.

Cornelison, F.S. and Arsenian, J. A study of the response of psychotic patients to photographic self-image experience. *Psychiatric Quarterly,* 1960, *34,* 1-8.

Danet, B.B. Self-confrontation in psychotherapy reviewed. *American Journal of Psychotherapy,* 1968, *22,* 245-258.

Duval, S., and Wicklund, R.A. *A theory of objective self-awareness.* New York: Academic Press, 1972.

Fitts, W.H. et al. Monograph series on the self concept. Available from Counselor Recordings and Tests, Box 6184, Acklen Station, Nashville, TN. 37212.

Fryrear, J.L. Videotape techniques for small training groups. In J.E. Jones and J.W. Pfeiffer (Eds), *The 1980 annual handbook for group facilitators.* San Diego, CA: University Associates, 1980.

Fryrear, J.L. and Fleshman, R. (Eds.), *Videotherapy in mental health.* Springfield, IL: Charles C Thomas, Publisher, 1981.

Fryrear, J.L., Kodera, T.L., and Kennedy, M.J. Self recognition ability in mentally retarded adolescents. *The Journal of Psychology,* 1981, *108,* 123-131.

Fryrear, J.L., and Nuell, L.R. *A photographic approach to self-concept modification in juvenile delinquents.* Technical report, Tennessee Law Enforcement Assistance Administration, 1973.

Fryrear, J.L., Nuell, L.R., and White, P. Enhancement of male juvenile delinquents' self concepts through photographed social interactions. *Journal of Clinical Psychology,* 1977, *33*(3), 833-838.

Hall, D.G. Photography as a learning experience in self-perception. *Phototherapy,* 1983, *3*(3).

Holzman, P.S., Rousey, C., and Snyder, C. On listening to one's own voice: Effects on psychophysiological responses and free associations. *Journal of Personality and Social Psychology,* 1966, *4,* 432-441.

Hung, J.H., and Rosenthal, T.L. Therapeutic videotaped playback. In J.L. Fryrear and R. Fleshman (Eds.), *Videotherapy in mental health.* Springfield IL: Charles C Thomas, Publisher, 1981.

Milford, S., Swank, P., and Fryrear, J.L. Enhancement of Self Esteem, Social Skills and Grooming in Institutionalized Adolescent Boys through Photography. Unpublished paper, University of Houston at Clear Lake City, 1981.

Miller, M.F. Responses of psychiatric patients to their photographed images. *Diseases of the Nervous System,* 1962, *23,* 196-198.

Pollack, M., Karp., E., Kahn, R.L., and Goldfarb, A.I. Perception of self in institutionalized aged subjects: I. Response patterns to mirror reflections. *Journal of Gerontology,* 1962, *17,* 405-408.

Rogers, C.R. A theory of therapy, personality, and interpersonal relationships, as developed in the client-centered framework. In S. Koch (Ed.) *Psychology: A study of a science,* Vol. 3. New York: McGraw-Hill, 1959.

Spire, R.H. Photographic self image confrontation. *American Journal of Nursing,* 1973, *73*(7), 1207-1210.

Vardell, M., McClellan, L., and Fryrear, J.L. A structured group phototherapy program and its use with adjudicated adolescent girls. *Phototherapy.* 1982, *3*(2).

Wicklund, R.A. Objective self-awareness: In L. Berkowitz (Ed.), *Advances in experimental social psychology,* Vol. 8. New York: Academic Press, 1975.

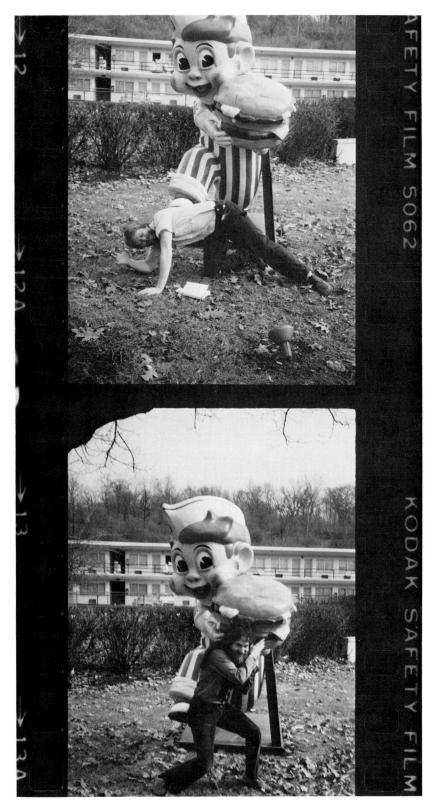

Photo by David A. Krauss

Chapter 6

The Psychological Niche: The Auto-Photographic Study of Self-Environment Interaction

ROBERT C. ZILLER, BRETT RORER, JEANNE COMBS AND DOUGLAS LEWIS

ONE of the main objectives of social science is to increase understanding of ourselves and significant others within an environmental setting. Understanding in contrast to knowing is a continuous phenomenological process, and is presumed to develop optimally when a variety of communication media are used. The present approach to understanding is phenomenological in that the perceiver is perceived through photographs *by* the perceiver rather than simply *of* the perceiver in an environment selected by the perceiver rather than by the observer. Through photography the person may show more than he/she can tell, and in the ensuing process of self-disclosure and self-understanding come to recognize the potential for change within the self-other environment ecosystem (the psychological niche).

Interpersonal understanding demands that one person consider everything in the environment of the other from the other's point of view with the intention of becoming more aware of, sensitized to, and realizing the uniqueness of the other. The essence of interpersonal understanding is other-realization.

Understanding and knowing the other are distinctly disparate (see Pelz, 1974). Knowing is somewhat impersonal, even distant, and in a context restricting change. Understanding, on the other hand, denotes something personal and unfinished within a continuously changing context. Knowing is a striving for certainty and categorization, whereas understanding is conditional, partial, and often open-ended. Understanding implies continuous search with an awareness of continuous change, including change in the observer.

Kelly (1955) has proposed that the other person's point of view can be operationalized in terms of that person's constructs, where constructs are schemas organizing the cognitive processes in the perception of others. In the present approach it is proposed that understanding emerges from the other person's view as this view is presented through the individual's self, social, and environmental orientations. These orientations are derived from images which

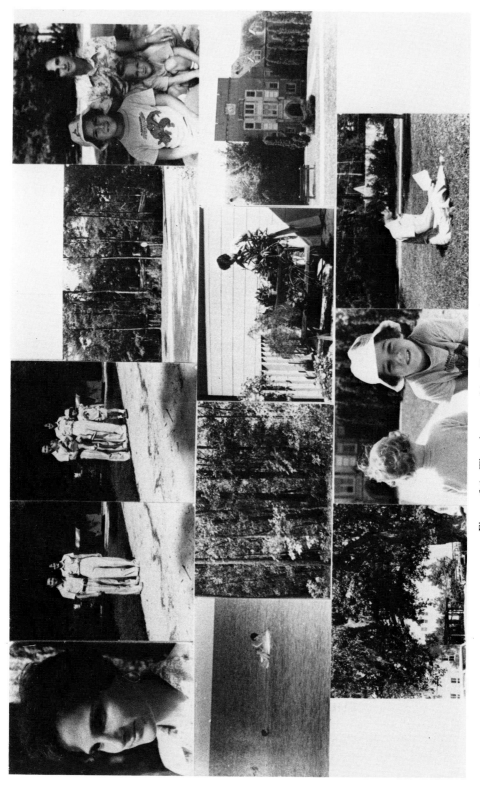

Figure 6-1. The photographic self-concept of a married woman.

are described by asking the person whom we are in the process of understanding to take a set of photographs that tell something about themselves (see Figure 6-1). Using the medium of images, the self-concept of the individual is described in terms of orientations as shown on film. The orientations are indications of the meaning of the self, but the self-concept also is associated with the selection of orientations. It is in the association between the self-concept and orientations that understanding of the person emerges.

Orientations are points of personal reference in the environment which render the situation meaningful and under the control of the individual. The individual scans the environment and structures it in terms of a set of objects of orientation (see Parsons & Shils, 1951, pp. 4-5). These objects are either social (individual actors or collectives) or nonsocial (physical objects or accumulated cultural resources). The orientation process entails selection of various objects through cognitive discrimination and the set of orientations represented as images describes the psychological niche for the actor.

The psychological niche that includes self-defining objects, persons and symbols serve as a source of self-reinforcement and reaffirmation of the self. The process is somewhat like looking into a mirror to reestablish contact with the somatic self. Selected objects, persons, and symbols in the person's environment serve to reaffirm the self and provide an environment which is meaningful or not alien. It is assumed that persons do not simply accept the environment as given, but create or influence the environment cognitively. Since the environmental field is vastly greater than a person can process or attend to, the individual is required to simplify the potential array of stimuli. The information reduction process begins with selective attention guided by self-schemas (Bartlett, 1932; Kelly, 1955). The individual scans the environment and attends to those aspects that are self-relevant. Those aspects of the environment attended, in turn, provide information about the self-schemas since the selection process is guided by a self-framework. Together, the orientations and the self-schemas indicated by the orientations provide the base for personal understanding.

Orientations and the schemas reflected in orientations provide a degree of personal control as opposed to environmental control. The individual does not respond directly to the environment as it is presented, but responds to those aspects of the environment that are deemed relevant to the self system. Thus, the psychological niche is a set of images of the individual's orientations that serve as a control mechanism through the process of self-affirmation. Finally, it is proposed that understanding of the individual will be improved through depiction of the psychological niche.

THE PHOTOGRAPHIC METAPHOR

Understanding begins with an effort to clarify the meaning. In this interpretative process the stimulus is often transformed using another domain of construction, an alternative frame of reference or language system to bear upon a set of observations. Indeed this is fundamental to the scientific approach, for example, the use of the model of an atom (Levy, 1963, p. 7). This juxtaposition of the elements into another framework, often a personal framework, stimulates cognitive process such as information search, comparison and contrast, and creativity. In the process personal meaning evolves. The cognitive processes lead to a unique interpretation by the individual within a personally constructed system. Often these interpretations are accompanied by images that are significant for the individual and help to integrate and assimilate the new concepts. This search for understanding through transformation to another domain describes the function of metaphor.

The study of metaphor dates back to Aristotle and has recently attracted the attention of psychologists (Billou, 1977; Ortony & Reynolds, 1978). Essentially metaphor depicts one thing in terms of another. It is essentially useful for the communication of things that cannot (or could not) be literally expressed or where the meaning must be construed rather than "read off" (Ortony & Reynolds, 1978, p. 2). It assumes that language is a creative activity rather than a computerized process. In this way metaphors can provide a different way of seeing the world and the articulation of new ideas.

Thus, Petrie (1979) proposes that the principal function of metaphor is to permit the understanding of new concepts by an iterative process from the more familiar metaphorical vehicle. It is a bridge between the known and the unknown through the use of ostensive reference. Perhaps this explains in part why metaphor is the medium for understanding by children.

Yet, the metaphor as studied to date emphasizes verbal communication, which may be the preferred representational system for a given group of persons (see Worth, 1974). Indeed, very often the metaphoric elements are mediated by images. The lesser known element of the metaphor evokes an image, which is then described verbally. In a sense, a most significant step in metaphoric communication is ignored because of the difficulty of studying images and the relative ease of analyzing the verbal response. The ease of analysis, however, may mask the questions of the validity of verbal responses. Do the subjective word labels mean what the investigator thinks they mean? Kelly (1955, p. 268) suggests that if a test "can be arranged to produce a kind of protocol which can be subjected to a meaningful analysis, independent of words, we shall have made great progress toward a better understanding" of the person. "We know more than we can tell" (Polanyi, 1966, p. 4) at least verbally; but through photographic communication, we may experience more than we know (see Pelz, 1974, p. 93). It is proposed here that photographic metaphor possesses many of these qualifications. Here the target system which is to be understood is new and abstract (Who are you?) and the base system in terms of which the target is described is familiar and perhaps visualizable (see

Gentner, 1980). The base system analogous to the target (Who are you?) is a series of photographs.

The resulting connections between the target, "Who are you?" (see Kuhn 1960), and the base, a set of photographs, may be called an "expressive metaphor" as opposed to an "explanatory metaphor." In the former value is placed on richness as opposed to clarity and consistency. The approach to photographic metaphor follows.

Auto-Photography

In the photographic approach to orientations (Ziller & Smith, 1977; Combs & Ziller, 1977), the subject is provided with a Kodak Instamatic® camera and twelve-exposure film and the following instructions:

> We want you to describe to yourself how you see yourself. To do this we would like you to take (or have someone else take) twelve photographs that tell who you are. These photographs can be of anything just as long as they tell something about who you are. You should not be interested in your skill as a photographer. Keep in mind that the photographs should describe who you are as you see yourself. When you finish you will have a book about yourself that is made up of only twelve photographs. Remember, these photographs are to simply tell something about you as you see yourself.

Among the first to use the "Who are you?" approach were Bugental and Zelen (1950). They merely provided the respondent with a blank piece of paper and asked him/her to give three answers to the question, "Who are you?" These answers were then classified by mention of name, status characteristics, affective quality, and the like.

Several advantages are inherent in the approach. Respondents are able to represent themselves in any frameworks they please; the approach is simple, and there is a quality of rich revealingness about the self-representation. Some of the same qualities are preserved by substituting photographs (by a non-sophisticated photographer) for words in response to "Who are you?" and at the same time some of the shortcomings of verbal responses are avoided. In addition, the photographic, nonverbal approach requires gross information reduction, is phenomenological, and may be the preferred representational system for subjects with communication handicaps.

The present approach builds on the pioneering work of Worth (see Gross, 1980 for a review). Worth, however used movies which provide a super-abundance of data rendering analysis difficult. Worth and Adair (1972), for example, asked Navajo Indians to shoot and edit movies about subjects of their own choosing. This approach is described by Worth (1961, p. 3) as a bio-documentary which he defines as ". . . a film made by a person to show how he feels about himself and his world. It is a subjective way of showing what the objective world that a person sees is really like. . . . In addition . . . it often captures feelings and reveals values, attitudes, and concerns that lie beyond the conscious control of the maker." The approach is seen by Worth as paralinguistics, which makes it easier for persons to talk to us (1966, p. 19).

The photographic self-concept only provides the starting point, however, for the more basic concern, orientation. By focusing on the self-concept, an affective and motivational component is introduced which personalizes the task, leading to more meaningful content. The study of orientations becomes the study of perceptions outside the laboratory, involving content meaningful to the subject and selected by the subject from a wide range of alternatives. An action component is introduced by requiring the subject to find the appropriate environment, to focus on the section of it which serves as the basis of the nonverbal message, and to make a decision by opening the camera shutter.

Content Analysis

The content analysis of the sets of photographs follows and extends the procedures used in earlier research with the "Who are you?" approach (Kuhn & McPartland, 1954) and the classic approaches to dream analysis (Hall & Van DeCastle, 1966). Consistent with theory of orientations, the content analysis involves the environmental, social and self constructs.

THE PSYCHOLOGICAL NICHE OF COUNSELEES[1]

The first study was designed to enhance understanding of counselees by the counselor as well as by the counselee through the photographic depiction of the counselee's psychological niche.

Rogers (1951) viewed the task of counseling as the expansion of self-awareness by enabling the client to experience himself or herself more fully in the present. Rogers emphasized the importance of the counselor's ability to perceive the internal reference of each client. Without this empathic understanding, it is proposed that the client will remain unaware of his present organismic experience.

Jourard (1964) points to the importance of self-disclosure to significant others as a means of experiencing the self. He discussed the ability to self-disclose as a fundamental concept for client and counselor in order to help the client move toward a healthy self-concept. It is proposed that the counseling process is facilitated if the counselor can experience the phenomenal field of the client.

The proposals by Rogers and Jourard are readily assimilated within the framework involving the psychological niche where the perception of the "internal reference of each client" as well as experiencing "the phenomenal field of

[1]This study is a reinterpretation of a study reported by Combs and Ziller (1977).

the client" both readily translate to the orientations of the client.

Method

Subjects

University students (N = 22) participated as volunteers in the study. There were eleven students (five females and six males) with a mean age of twenty years who were counselees at the university clinic, and eleven students matched for age and sex.were members of an introductory social psychology class. The counseling subjects were all the clients of a single counselor during two college terms, excluding those whose stated purpose was vocational counseling and three subjects who declined.

Each person was provided with an Instamatic camera and a twelve-picture roll of black-and-white film.

Procedure

The following instructions were given to each student:

> Place yourself in this situation. You are sending a series of twelve photographs one by one through the mail to someone you will meet in two weeks. You want to give a true impression of yourself. I want you to take, or have taken, a series of photographs. I also want to know the order in which you plan to send them, so when they are developed, number them from 1 to 12, marking the first photograph to be sent with a 1. The subject of the photographs can be anything you choose, as long as you think it is communicating something about who you are. I am not interested in your photographic skills. The photographs are only a way of communicating nonverbally who you are.

Content Analysis

The content analysis of the sets of photographs follows and extends the procedures used in earlier research with the verbal "Who are you?" approach by Kuhn and McPartland (1954), the classic approaches to dream analysis (Hall & Van DeCastle, 1966), and the "vidistic" approach by Worth (1966). The evolving coding categories are presented in Table 6-I.

Each student in the counseling and noncounseling situation discussed their photographs with one of the authors. In the counseling situation the photographic self-concept was introduced in the third or fourth session, and the photographs were used subsequently as a technique for clarification of the self-concept.

The photographs taken by the counseled group (see Figure 6-2 for an exam-

Table 6-I

Client and Non-Client Difference in Self Presentation

	Client Group	Non-Client Group	X^2	Fisher's Exact Test	p.
Family	.36	.00	4.88		.05
Self	.54	1.00		.0175	
Other Person	.90	1.00	1.05		NS
Past	.36	.00		.045	
Self and Other	.18	.45	1.88		NS
Activities	.27	.81	6.6		.025
Animals	.27	.36	.20		NS
Books	.27	.72	4.56		.05
Significant Other	.45	.72	1.7		NS

Note.--The significance of the differences were tested by chi-square for all categories with the exceptions of "self" and "past." In the latter cases the test used was Fisher's exact test (Hays, 1973, p. 738) because of the low expected frequencies.

ple) were compared with those taken by the control group (see Figure 6-1 for an example) using ten categories. These same categories were used in earlier research by the first author following a phenomenological analysis of ninety sets of photographic self-concepts of college students (see Ziller & Smith, 1977).

RESULTS

The results of the chi-square and Fisher's exact test (Hays, 1973, p. 738) analyses are presented in Table 6-I. Each group was given a percentage score for each category according to the number of photographs in which they had included pictures of self, pictures of self and others, pictures of others, pictures of family, pictures from the past, pictures of activities, hedonic tone (percent of photographs involving people where at least one person is smiling), pictures of books (earlier research by Ziller and Smith in 1977 showed a significant positive correlation between orientation toward books and scholastic achievement), pictures of significant others (friends, spouse), and pictures of animals. If the subject included one or more photographs involving books, a score of 1 was assigned. If no books were included, a score of 0 was assigned. The photographs were scored independently by the authors. The *two* scores were consistent 95 percent of the time. Inconsistencies were reconciled through discussion. The activities category presented the only disagreement. Those photographs classified as activity pictures involving sports, musical instruments, chess, parties, sewing, painting, cooking, biking, and gardening. The significance of the differences were tested by chi-square for all categories with the exceptions of the self and past. In the latter cases, the test used was the Fisher's exact test (Hays, 1973, p. 738) because of the low expected frequencies.

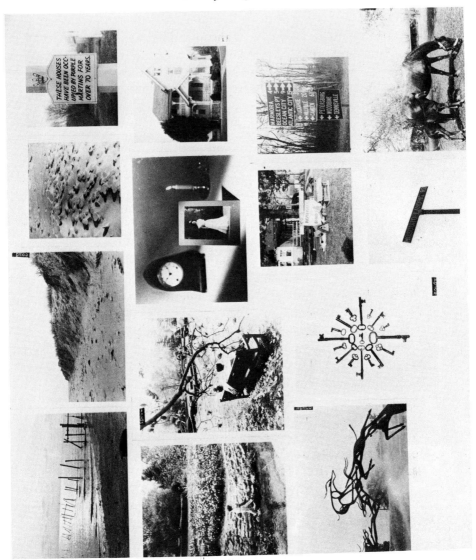

Figure 6-2. The photographic self-concept of a woman in transition.

The counseled groups' photographs were significantly different from the non-counseled groups' photographs on five of the nine dimensions at the .05 level of confidence. The counseled group presented significantly more pictures of the past and of their families. They presented significantly fewer photographs of themselves, their activities, their books, and their photographs showed lower hedonic tone.

Discussion

The study explored nine facets of photographic self-presentation. The data illustrate that students in counseling present different facets of self-image than do other students. Half of the counseled group included photographs of themselves. In contrast, the nonclient group presented photographs of themselves in every instance. This could be interpreted in several ways. First, the client group expressed verbally a feeling of self-consciousness and inadequacy about their personal appearance. This feeling was not voiced in the nonclient group. Thus a lack of self-esteem is indicated among the client group of students who do not accept their physical appearance. The photographic approach to the self-concept facilitates this communication.

Two other facets of client self-concept that were significantly different from the nonclient group were the choice of family photographs and photographs from the past. In the nonclient group, not one person included any photographs in either of these categories in his or her photographic self-concept. The client group may have been experiencing difficulties in defining themselves in terms other than that of a family self-identity; that is, they may have been experiencing difficulty in making the transition from the family setting. Laing and Esterson (1964) have discussed the problems that may develop within an individual if they cannot find a sense of self outside the family nexus.

A need to return to the past may characterize the individual in transition. Mueller (1973) has noted that a client who is experiencing conflict may seek a less conflicted mode of experiencing such as reliving past conflicts with others.

In contrast to the emphasis on the family and the past by clients, lack of emphasis was observed concerning activities and books. Only 27 percent of the client group included these categories in their photographic self-concept. The nonclient group included activities and books 81 percent of the time. Subjects in the nonclient group described their self-images in terms of activities such as swimming, tennis, biking, and studying. The client group presented remarkably few activities of this kind as being associated with the self-image. Because a college environment usually included a variety of these activities, these data suggest that the client group is alienated. Perhaps, again, these clients are experiencing difficulty in transition from the home to the college environment, or more generally, the client group is under conflict and stress that leads to a more closed and less active participation in their present environment. Some turn to the past for orientation. For the present, all have recourse to a counselor. Perhaps it is the future that poses one of the significant difficulties, or a time orientation in general. The counselee has experienced a discontinuity among life events (loss of a close friend, for example) that renders the future extraordinarily uncertain. Thus, the task of counseling is to reestablish a relationship among the client's past, present, and future.

The significant differences in the photographic self-concepts of clients and controls attest to the validity of the approach and its broad utility as a research technique. The photographic self-concept is a nonverbal approach that enables others to perceive the perceiver, to see others as others see themselves. It can lead to an improved understanding of a wide variety of groups and persons, as has previously been demonstrated (Ziller & Smith, 1977). In addition, however, the utility of the approach in counseling is suggested.

In one case, for example, the client seemed to present many of the photographs common to the control group. A closer inspection of the photographs showed no books, no photographs of his wife, and a number of photographs from the past including a photograph of his mother and grandmother whom he visited weekly. The emerging theme was difficulty with the present social environment and an attempt to emphasize continuity with the past. Using the photographs as stimulus materials with the client as a partner in the inquiry can lead to increased empathic understanding through the delineation of the psychological niche of the client.

The psychological niche takes into account the person-environment interaction. The auto-photographic approach to the study of the psychological niche compels consideration of the environment in understanding persons and imposes ecological validity.

By definition, however, the psychological niche is interactional. Orientations emerge both from personal schemas and from the characteristics of the environment. Thus, the counselee selects the orientations to the past, limited activities, and reduced hedonic tone, but then the selected orientations (the psychological niche) become the special environment of the individual and reflexively limits the behavior of the counselee, thereby creating a spiraling effect in the existing directions of development (a self-fulfilling prophecy). In a sense, the psychological niche becomes a social trap (Platt, 1973). The niche is created in an effect to achieve a degree of personal control, but the niche also limits adaptability to the environment that the person must enter eventually. The quest for equanimity in the immediate environment retards the transition to the imminent environment.

A large number of questions remain to be answered. How can the photographic self-concept approach be used in a counseling setting? How are the counselor's perception of the client and the client's perception of the counselor altered when the photographic self-concept is employed? What are the characteristics of clients who avoid using the approach? Under what circumstances is communication between the client and the counselor facilitated through the photographic self-concept approach?

It is clear, however, that the approach has several advantages. The client is able to represent himself/herself in any framework he/she pleases; the approach is simple; the approach is creative rather than reactive; there is a quality of "rich revealingness" about the self-presentation, deriving, in part, from the unintentional information in addition to the intentional information, and at the same time some of the usual shortcomings of verbal responses are avoided. As Kelly suggests (1955), "If a test can be arranged to produce a kind of protocol that can be subjected to a meaningful analysis, independent of words, we shall have made progress toward a better understanding of the client's personal constructs" (p. 268).

THE PSYCHOLOGICAL NICHE OF JUVENILE DELINQUENTS[2]

Explanations of juvenile delinquency are many and varied (Matza, 1969), yet unconvincing. The present study was designed to develop a better understanding of the person in question from that person's point of view as he/she describes his/her orientations which define that psychological niche.

Method

Subjects

The comparison groups comprised thirty-five male students in two alternative education settings and forty-four male students from two public school settings. The students in the alternative school settings were assigned to the schools because of a wide range of antisocial behaviors requiring the involvement of criminal justice officers. Other than in the school setting, however, the juvenile delinquents were not restricted and all lived with their families. The subjects in the control group were volunteers from social science classes in two public schools. The racial composition of the two groups was the same, 68 percent white and 32 percent black. The age range was eleven to seventeen years with a mean of fifteen in both groups.

Procedure

Again the subjects were provided with an Instamatic camera with a twelve-shot load of film along with the following instructions (somewhat altered for the sake of improved clarity):

> We want you to describe to yourself how you see yourself. To do this we would like you to take (or have someone else take) twelve photographs that

---

[2]This study is a reinterpretation of a study by Ziller and Lewis (1981).

tell who your are. These photographs can be of anything just as long as they tell something about who you are. You should not be interested in your skill as a photographer. Keep in mind that the photographs should describe who you are as you see yourself. When you.finish you will have a book about yourself that is made up of only twelve photographs.

Content Analysis

The content analysis of the sets of photographs follows and extends the procedures used in the previous study. Consistent with the theory of orientations, the content analysis involves environmental, social, and self constructs. Inclusion of "self" could not be coded because the subjects were not known to the coders. Social orientation was coded as the percent of total number of photographs in which at least one person was shown (earlier research by the senior author shows that shy persons include fewer photographs of others). An example of an environmental construct is aesthetic orientation, the percent of photographs focusing upon the sky, water, flowers, works of art, and the like. Previous research demonstrated a significant correlation ($r = .34$, $p < .05$) between aesthetic orientation and aesthetic values as measured by the Vernon-Allport-Lindsey Study of Values. Other coded orientations which emerged and were identified by a preliminary scan of the photographs included: school (whether or not the subject's photographs included at least one photograph that focused upon a school building), home (whether or not the subject's photographs included at least one photograph that focused upon a home), family (whether or not the subject's photographs included at least one photograph that included a member of his family). The sets of photographs were coded independently by two raters and discussed to agreement in the few cases where discrepancies occurred.

Results

Juvenile delinquents in comparison with the control groups were far less likely to show aesthetic orientation (11% versus 45%, $X^2 = 10.7$, $p < .01$) and academic orientation or books (3% versus 11% but the frequencies were too small to test statistically). Moreover, the delinquents showed photographs of a school less frequently (11% versus 66%, $X^2 = 13.8$, $p < .0001$), as well as photographs of a home (51% versus 66%, NS). The delinquents, however, tended to show photographs including people more frequently (68% versus 39%, $X^2 = 3.08$, $p < .01$).

Discussion

Through the set of orientations that describe the psychological niche, a new basis for understanding delinquency emerges. It is seen that the psychological niche of the control group includes home, school, and aesthetics. In contrast, the psychological niche of the delinquent includes peers and smiling persons.

The psychological niche is developed by the individual to serve as an area of self-affirmation and reinforcement, and provides a region over which the individual possesses some degree of control. For the nondelinquents, that region of security is defined as social institutions (home and school) and socially approved readily available source of self-reinforcement, aesthetic orientation. In contrast, delinquent youths' psychological niche is defined in terms of peers and smiling persons. The environment created by delinquents may serve as a substitute for the environment that is not available to him/her because of a different personal history where the usual institutional affiliations have not been found adequately rewarding. An orientation to peers provides the niche required for self-affirmation and personal control. The environment created by delinquents now interacts with the individual and reinforces behaviors that are outside the field of the institutional setting (home and school). The mere separation establishes the basis of a conflict between peers and institutional settings where members of the separate groups now tend to reinforce members of their special group in preference to other persons (Tajfel, 1981). This exclusive reinforcement tendency leads to further exclusion and distance and the exclusion is attributed to irreconcilable differences, which exacerbate the association between peer groups and the usual sources of socialization.

The conflict begins with the exclusion of delinquents from social institutions and the separate inclusion in peer groups. Improvement of the dilemma probably may be signaled by attempts at integrating the two separate groups.

The conflict described here emerged from the attempt to better understand delinquent youth through visual communication. But understanding implies a process. The visual communication of intentional and unintentional elements in the photographs only provides the data in first approximation. Understanding requires a commitment to continuously strive to comprehend and to avoid the sense of knowing. Knowing suggests a conclusion; understanding is openended and thereby more hopeful.

SELF-OTHER UNDERSTANDING THROUGH
AUTO-PHOTOGRAPHIC FEEDBACK

An approach to self-other understanding has been proposed through autophotographic metaphor. In a sense, the approach derives from symbolic interaction (see Meltzer, Petras, & Reynolds, 1975). The individual constructs a set of photographs concerning the self, and these photographs are symbols to which the individual reacts through assimilation and accommodation. In this process the individual comes to perceive the construct system (here, psychological niche) of the self and self-understanding is enhanced. When this process takes place in association with a therapist, the therapist facilitates self-understanding by viewing the frozen images of the client's self mirrored in the photographic array. The process is one of nonverbal self-disclosure to the self with the aid of a professional guide.

The therapist serves as a nonthreatening audience. Thereby the subject examines public reaction to the self as disclosed nonverbally. The process is one of desensitization through images to the self as portrayed.

In addition to imparting an audience effect, the therapist helps to prevent the client from simply running circles around the self. Alone with the set of photographs portraying the self, the client often reports circular, redundant, undirected interactions. This tendency is avoided simply because the therapist serves as a recorder (in a symbolic sense) and the client with the aid of the therapist is guided toward a more systematic and directed self-analysis and self-understanding.

Simply by returning to the topic of the depicted psychological niche, self-understanding is facilitated by the addition of time considerations. Understanding emerges over time. It is the function of the therapist to provide the structure for the client to return and return again to the photographic niche as portrayed. Even in the process of repeatedly returning to the subject of the self, the very process indicates nonverbally that self becomes more understandable but is never known.

The therapist and client together explore the nature of the client's psychological niche. Because the client is most familar with the portrayed environment, the counselor and client share control of the therapeutic process, and, indeed, the counselor is required to listen, because the therapy, in a sense, takes place outside the office of the therapist in the client's domain as portrayed in the photographs.

As the client and counselor examine the psychological niche of the client, the components of the self-social environment emerge and the sources of security are revealed; persons, objects, aesthetics, the self, selected activities, and related environments. When the set of photographs is presented as a complete array before the client, the client is sometimes confronted with the special nature of the environment which he/she has created (see Figure 6-4). Here the counselor and client together may explore why the client must at least share the responsibility for the environmental context of the self, and more than that, recognize how the environment, which he/she is partially responsible for creating, in turn imposes itself on the client by restricting alternatives. Essentially the client comes to discover that he/she has created a psychological niche which creates the self, in turn.

The final phase in the process is designed to develop a strategy for altering the psychological niche. Thus, the person whose psychological niche is shown in Figure 6-3 was shy. When it evolved that no persons were portrayed (at least in any proximity), and the stark emptiness of the niche became apparent to the client, the client initiated a resocialization program and actively created an environment which, in interaction, created through extended alternatives a

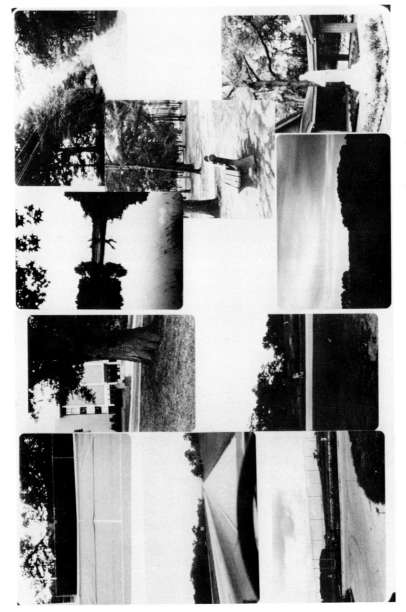

Figure 6-3. The photographic self-concept of a shy college student.

broader range of orientations.

Auto-photography provides a feedback to clients about their self-environment interaction. The feedback is in the form of images which for most clients are quickly assimilated and arranged to form a self-gestalt. In this form the individual is often capable of intrapersonal communication about self-environment interactions and the potential and desire for change.

Americkaner, Schauble, and Ziller (1981) have noted other counseling procedures involving auto-photography. What a client does not include in the photos may be critical such as the exclusion of the self and other people by the shy person previously discussed.

Essentially, however, auto-photography is simply a nonverbal approach to communication, and the nonverbal approach is easily expanded and fashioned for the central area of concern for the client. For example, under conditions of marriage counseling, at an appropriate point in the counseling process it may be helpful to ask both parties to take or have taken six photographs in response to each of the following questions:

Who am I?
Who are you? (spouse)
Who are we? (self and spouse)

The nonverbal responses provided information about co-orientations that may provide the basis of mutual understanding.

Newcombe (1968, p. 55) has proposed that communication among persons enables two or more individuals to maintain simultaneous orientation (co-orientation) toward one another as communication and toward objects of communication. Moreover, the more intense one person's concern for another, the more sensitive he is likely to be to the other's orientations to objects in the environment. Thus, members of a social group may be expected to be oriented toward objects in the environment and toward other persons in the group oriented toward those same objects.

An approach to marital counseling that involves sets of orientations of the man-woman dyad begins with the triad of questions presented above and the dyad's photographic responses. Commonalities among orientations are cited by the members of the dyad and differences are discussed to the members' satisfaction. Validity for the basis of the approach was provided by an unpublished study (Ricketson, 1981) which shows a significant correlation ($r = .39$, $p < .05$) between co-orientation of values portrayed by three photographs in answer to the question "What is important to you?" and ratings of marital satisfaction by married women.

A second example of ad hoc photographic tasks that are designed to respond to the demands of the particular client involves a client with chronic back pain. The therapy process was hampered by the client's unwillingness to communicate verbally. In order to facilitate communication, the client was given the following three questions in sequence to which he was to respond nonverbally with six photographs to each question:

> My home and neighborhood is?
> Who am I?
> What makes me feel good?

The sequence of questions was designed first to acquaint the client with the approach with a low threat question. The second question again enables the subject to describe the psychological niche. The third question and responses were critical, however. Through the question the client is induced to begin a positive reorientation program. By focusing on sources of positive reinforcement in the environment and supporting this orientation in discussing the images with the client, the basis for the development of a more supporting psychological niche is established.

Essentially, this later approach may be described as a cognitive-behavioral intervention (see Kendall & Hollon, 1979) where positive imagery is a source of self-reinforcement. Here it is assumed that the depressed individual's environment is a self-fulfilling prophecy. The environment (or psychological niche) of the depressed person facilitates continued depression. In order to break the self-defeating interaction, a cognitive restructuring is developed through photographic images. The client is directed toward facets of his/her environment that are in the positive direction. Viewing these areas (and even conjuring up the images) is reinforcing and the image behavior is repeated until it becomes a part of the psychological niche.

In a sense the question, "What makes me feel good?" leads to photographic responses that indicate the value orientations of the client. A more direct approach to value orientations that has been developed (Rorer & Ziller, 1982) involves the question, "What the good life means" and photographic responses. Again, however, there are advantages to developing a series of questions that are responsive to the characteristics of the special client.

RESTRUCTURING THE PSYCHOLOGICAL NICHE

The therapy process involving auto-photography is a reflexive approach that begins with a theory of the self set in images. The theory incorporates a uniquely heavy emphasis on the environment in interaction with the person. The self-environment interaction is abstracted in terms of orientations, and the set of orientations (the psychological niche) is at once the source of stability but also the focus for change for persons under conditions of stress. In fact, the effectiveness of the change may be indicated by changes in the psychological niche over time, and the evaluation of the change becomes part of the therapeutic process by using pre-post auto-photographic studies followed by reactions to both sets of photographs.

The restructuring of the psychological niche may take any of a variety of directions, including expansion of the range of orientations with regard to shy persons to less emphasis on given facets of the psychological niche such as the self for self-centered persons. The restructuring may also focus on the time orientation, the orientation toward the past, present, or future; for example the representation of parents from the past to friends in the immediate environment for persons under conditions of counseling in an academic environment.

The restructuring process begins with self-disclosure through auto-photography and the development of an awareness of the psychological niche depicted and the negotiation with the therapist about the outcomes in terms of losses and gains following the course of change.

Overview

An approach to the study and use of the iconic communication of person-people-place interaction has been described. The approach placed the individual in an environmental context and the resulting portrayal of the psychological niche indicates the individual's critical domain as outlined by the set of orientations. This domain is created by the person, but the domain in turn limits the behavior of the person. Thus, the person becomes controlled by his/her own attempts to control the environment. The psychological niche is the place where personal meanings dwell. Thus, in order to understand someone (including the self), the orientations and the pscyhological niche of the person must be described.

Understanding is a process, however, requiring time, multi-methods of communication and a phenomenological approach. By perceiving the perceiver the underlying orientations of the perceiver may be clarified, thereby providing the basis of understanding. But understanding is an endless process. In the process of understanding through auto-photography it is communicated nonverbally to the subject of understanding that it is indeed a process unlike the finality of knowing.

The unfolding process of understanding presents a climate of potential for change and is therefore an induction of hope. The study of the psychological niche through auto-photography is like holding a multifaceted mirror before the subject that includes a time factor ranging from the past, from which the self evolves, to the future, to which the individual is making a transition. Persons are defined by their orientations. Thus, understanding begins with a person's description of his/her orientations and works back to the person or the perceiver.

REFERENCES

Americkaner, N., Schauble, P, & Ziller, R.C. The use of photographs in personal counseling. *Personnel and Guidance Journal*, 1980, *59*, 68-73.
Bandura, A. Self-efficacy: Toward a unifying theory of behavioral changes. *Psychological Review*, 1977, *84*, 191-215.
Bartlett, F.C. *Remembering*. Cambridge: Cambridge University Press, 1932.

Billow, R.M. Metaphor: A review of psychological literature, *Psychological Bulletin*, 1977, *84*, 81-92.

Bugental, J.F.T., & Zelen, S.L. Investigations into the "self-concept": I The W-A-Y technique. *Journal of Personality*, 1950, *18*, 488-498.

Combs, J. & Ziller, R.C. The photographic self-concept of counselors. *Journal of Counseling Psychology*, 1977, *24*, 452-455.

Gentner, D. On the development of metaphor processing. *Child Development*, 1977, *48*, 1034-1039.

Gross, L. Sol Worth and the study of visual communications, *Visual Communication*, 1980, *6*, 2-19.

Hall, C.S. & Van De Castle, R.V. *The content analysis of dreams*. Englewood Cliffs, N.J.: Prentice-Hall, 1966.

Hays, W.L. *Statistics for the social sciences*. New York: Holt, Rinehart & Winston, 1973.

Jourard, S.M. *The transparent self*. New York: Van Nostrand, 1964.

Kanfer, F.H. & Karaly, P. Self-control: A behaviorist's excursion into the lions den. *Behavior Therapy*, 1972, *3*, 398-416.

Kelly, G.A. *The psychology of personal constructs*. New York: Norton, 1955.

Kendall, P.C. & Hollon, S.C. *Cognitive-behavioral interventions*. New York: Academic Press, 1979.

Kuhn, M.H. Self attitudes by age, sex, and professional training. *Sociological Quarterly*, 1960, *1*, 39-55.

Kuhn, M.H., & McPartland, T.S. An empirical investigation of self-attitudes. *American Sociological Review*, 1954, *19*, 68-76.

Laing, R.D., & Esterson, A. *Sanity, madness and the family: Families of schizophrenics*. London: Tavistock Publications, 1964.

Levy, L.H. *Psychological interpretation*. New York: Holt, Rinehart, & Winston, 1963.

Matza, D. *Becoming deviant*. Englewood Cliffs, NJ: Prentice-Hall, 1969.

Meltzer, B.N., Petras, J.W. & Reynolds, L.T. *Symbolic interactionism: Genesis, varieties and criticism*. London: Pautledge, 1975.

Mueller, W.J. Avenues to understanding: *The dynamics of therapeutic interaction*. New York: Appleton-Century-Crofts, 1973.

Newcombe, T.M. The prediction of interpersonal attraction, *American Psychologist*, 1956, *11*, 575-586.

Ortony, A. & Reynolds, R.E. Metaphor theoretical and empirical research, *Psychological Bulletin*, 1978, *85*, 919-943.

Parsons, T. & Shils, E.A. *Toward a general theory of action*. Cambridge, Massachusetts: Harvard University Press, 1951.

Pelz, W. *The scope of understanding in sociology*. London: Routledge & Kegan Paul, 1974.

Petrie, H. Metaphor and learning. In *Metaphor and thoughts,* A. Ortony (Ed.). Cambridge: Cambridge University Press, 1979.

Platt, G. Social traps, *American Psychologist*, 1973, *28*, 641-651.

Rorer, B. & Ziller, R.C. Value orientations among Polish and American students. Unpublished Masters thesis, University of Florida, Gainesville, Florida, 1982.

Ricketson, H. Congruence of marital satisfaction and values. Unpublished Honor thesis:- University of Florida, 1981.

Rogers, C.R. *Client centered therapy*. Boston: Houghton-Mifflin, 1951.

Tajfel, H. The psychological structures of intergroup relations. In J. Toffed (Ed.), *Differentiation between social groups: Studies in social psychology of intergroup relations*. London: Academic Press, European Monographs in Social Psychology, 1981.

Worth, S. Film as non-art: an approach to the study of film. *The American Scholar*, 1966, *35*, 422-334.

Worth, S. Public administration and the documentary film, *Journal of Municipal Association for Management and Administration*, 1964.

Worth, S. Seeing metaphor as caricature. *New Literary History*, 1974, *6*, 195-209.

Worth, S. & Adair, J. *Through Navajo eyes.* Bloomington, Indiana: Indiana University Press, 1972.

Ziller, R.C. Psychology and photography. *The Photographer,* Fall 1975.

Ziller, R.C. & Lewis, D. Orientations: self, social, and environmental precepts through autophotography. *Personality and Social Psychology Bulletin,* 1981, 338-343.

Ziller, R.C. & Smith, D.E. A phenomenological utilization of photographs. *Journal of Phenomenological Psychology,* 1977, *7,* 172-185.

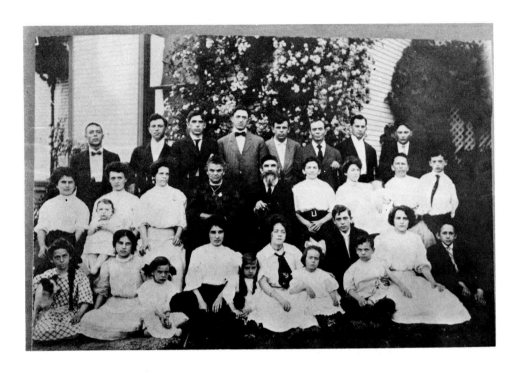

Photographer unknown. Collection of David A. Krauss.

Chapter 7

The Family Photo Album as Icon: Photographs in Family Psychotherapy

ALAN D. ENTIN

> As photographs are passed from hand to hand, generation to generation, they take on the patina of relationship and the human touch, and weave like a golden thread through time and the movement of human beings. The object becomes more than it is, something over and above its original form.
>
> William De Lappa, 1981

FAMILY PHOTO ALBUMS: ICONS OF THE FAMILY

FAMILY photographs are highly cherished, treasured objects, irreplaceable reminders of family, friends and experiences. They recall a person, a time, a place, a ceremony, an event. They are valued over and above the image and are imbued with special meanings. Those photographs that take on significance as "favorite photographs," are treasured for their visual and nonvisual, metaphoric, symbolic representations and remembrances. They become elevated to the status of an icon. They are records that contain the individual and collective history of the family and its members, reflecting the movement through time and space of the individuals that comprise the family. Family photographs give striking visual evidence of ancestors, and through their changing modes of dress and life-styles, of the traditions, values and ideals of the family over the generations. The albums testify to a sense of continuity for the family as a visual record of ancestors whose existence preceded the present generation and of images of family members that one day would be seen by generations who succeed the present generation. Observance of the rites of passage, ceremonies, significant family and social gatherings, holidays

This is to CAPITALLY acknowledge (punish) J.A. for his latest carryings on in his efforts to teach the author good English usage. I appreciate the critical reading of the manuscript by Phyllis C. Entin, M.A. I am deeply appreciative of the assistance provided by George Nan in preparing the photographs for publications, and I would like to thank Michael Crane for permission to reproduce his photograph/sculpture *Horizon Triangle*. I am grateful to the many individuals who contributed to my understanding of the family photo album as icon through their efforts at understanding their family systems.

117

and individuals included in the photographs provide further opportunity to examine and explore the family system. The photograph albums reflect how the family chooses to document its existence as a family. Since the camera can capture and preserve a "minislice" of family history, important questions are raised as to the meanings surrounding these activities, as well as the relationships and events selected to be permanent photographic images. The records form the history of the family and present a collective image of the family. The albums are documents that can be studied to learn about what this particular family values and what were its commonalities and differences with other families (Entin, 1982).

The family photographs are like totem poles (Entin, E., 1981), visual family trees pointing both to the past, where the family came from, "to learn lessons from the past" (Barrow, 1980, p. 35), and to learn where the family is going in the future. They are a form of communication addressing the question: What does it mean to be a person, a man, a woman, a child, in this family? Who, what, where, when and how events are selected to be photographed and included in the family album are significant facts about the family. Family albums reflect a continuation of generational rhythms in the family life cycle, presenting a recurring pattern of relationships linking people, the passage of time, and the organization of space far more systematically than is usually recognized. Family photographs and albums function as icons of the family reflecting the collective past, the symbols of attachment and connectedness to the traditions and ideals of the family, providing evidence of continuity in the present and pointing the way for the values in the future (Entin, 1981).

PHOTOGRAPHS IN FAMILY PSYCHOTHERAPY

There are many diverse ways that photographs and family albums have and can be used in individual and family psychotherapy. The multiplicity of creative approaches underscore the ubiquity of photographs and the profundity of visual images in our culture, perhaps in most cultures in our century, reflecting the tremendous technological advances in image making. Press the button, the storyteller does the rest. It only takes a few seconds and, with study, "understanding your family may be a snap" (Fenjves, 1981). However, to be able to look at photographs and family albums to learn about family relationships requires an understanding of family systems theory. I approach family photographs and albums within the theoretical framework provided by Bowen family systems theory. The principle that guides my thinking is "How can the concepts of family systems theory be operationalized and conveyed visually?" It is this approach which will be the subject of this chapter.

BOWEN FAMILY SYSTEMS THEORY AND THERAPY

Theory

Bowen family systems theory describes and conceptualizes the family relationship system and the variables that affect its changing patterns and processes over time. Physical, social and emotional dysfunctioning are symptoms of disturbance in the family emotional process. The theory deals with the facts (who, what, where, when and how) of the family. The important interlocking concepts include: (1) triangles; (2) nuclear family process (manifest through emotional distance, marital conflict, spouse dysfunction via emotional, physical or social symptoms), and/or impairment of children; (3) family projection process; (4) differentiation of self; (5) multigenerational transmission process; (6) emotional cutoff; (7) sibling position and (8) societal emotional process.

It is essential for the therapist to have the prerequisite skills, knowledge and training in the theoretical base before attempting to study photograph albums. Once the concepts are understood, ideas for their interpretation and translation into visual images will suggest themselves to the therapist. The application of the concepts to the observation of family albums are extensions of the theory. Although a detailed presentation of Bowen family systems theory is beyond the scope of this paper, several concepts of the theory will be presented as illustrative of ways they may be manifest or inferred in photographs. A more general theoretical discussion of the application of the theory to the study of photographs and family albums is presented in *Photo Therapy: Family Albums and Multigenerational Portraits* (Entin, 1980) and *Family Icons: Photographs in Family Therapy* (Entin, 1982). A more comprehensive exposition of family systems theory and psychotherapy can be obtained from the writings of Murray Bowen (1971, 1972, 1976), especially his book *Family Therapy in Clinical Practice* (1978), and "Family Systems Theory and Therapy" by Kerr (1981).

Training

In discussing the training of family systems therapists, Kerr describes two characteristics which interfere with therapeutic functioning: the therapist's (1) "intense urge to offer and adhere to explanations for things they do not really understand"; (2) the "tendency to intrude anxiously into emotionally charged problem situations" (1981, p. 226). In order to assist the family to control anxiety and be able to observe and think about the problems, the therapist must be in control of the therapist's own anxiety and thinking. Kerr states:

> we have tried to. . .keep(ing) the main emphasis on theory and the therapist's ability to avoid simplistic concepts and solutions to human problems. If a therapist can be clear that he or she can never have more than a very small percentage of answers, best called reasonably accurate assumptions based on current knowledge, this attitude will do more than anything else to help the problem family out of its own "fix-it" or "make-it-go-away" mentality into a more inquiring, contemplative mode.
>
> This training takes a long time because these urges are deep in people's emotional makeup and are particularly pronounced when they are anxious. It takes a long time to recognize and gain some control over this process within oneself.
>
> (1981, pp. 226-7)

This passage is particularly relevant when the therapist attempts to use photographs in family therapy. All too often it is assumed that "photographs in family therapy" merely means bringing photographs to a therapy session as a focus for discussion. Although such an approach may be interesting, arresting, occasionally "cathartic," or perhaps even "therapeutic," it is simply a technique. A technique that is not grounded in theory or that is utilized by an untrained therapist with a "fix-it" or "make-it-go-away" mentality, however, may compound the problem. From my perspective it is essential that the therapist have a solid theoretical background and training in the field so as to be able to "think systems." Then it becomes possible to read family photo albums in the language of family systems theory.

Therapy

The concepts of family systems theory determine the information to be gathered in family therapy sessions, especially during the early evaluation phase. Questions can be organized about the relationships in the family using the structure of the genogram (Entin, 1978, 1982). Information can be gathered about the history and course of the presenting problems, the history of the nuclear family and the history of the extended family of the husband and wife. Then the therapist and family can define an area for each family member to change in themselves in order to lower the level of anxiety in self and thereby control one's part in the emotional process.

As part of the process of differentiating self in the family and learning about the extended family of origin of each spouse, contact with parents, grandparents and other significant family members is necessary. Often presented as "I already know all about them" (fusion), or "I don't want to have anything to do with them" (emotional cutoff), an individual's reluctance to contact the family is a resistance to understanding and dealing with unresolved issues in current problems. One technique for dealing with this resistance is suggesting that it might be useful to look at family photographs with family as a way to facilitate entering and making contact with significant members of the family. Usually it is best accomplished individually with each parent (as well as other relatives), rather than with both together. This allows discussing each individual's point of view without getting involved in the family "togetherness" and therefore allowing more opportunity to work towards defining a self in relation to each parent. Thus, the experience has the twofold purpose of getting information about past generations (the extended family of origin over time as well as current multigenerational issues) and developing and maintaining relationships in the present. With this framework it actually may be unnecessary for family members to bring in and discuss photographs during a family psychotherapy session.

During psychotherapy sessions, the therapist's questions are designed to teach the concepts of family systems theory through relevant examples from the family history. It is intended that the family members become experts at understanding how their family works, e.g. how anxiety and symptoms affect the level of differentiation of family members and are projected onto the next generation via the multigenerational transmission process. The questions asked and information gathered during a family therapy session are those to be used while looking at family albums with one's own family. This includes details about the people, places and events in the photographs. The aim is to get a better reading on family members' relationships with one another.

The theory is a guide to think about the photographs: there are no direct translations or correspondences between the theory and the photographs. Similarly, "There is no generalized, one-to-one correspondence between what is present in the photograph and a fact or interpretation about this or any other family" (Entin, 1982, p. 219). Some concepts may be directly observed and some inferred, while others may not be capable of translation into physical or visual terms. While there are many clues and hypotheses generated by the theory, it is the individual who must use the opportunity of reviewing photographs with the family to raise questions and start discussions. Their examinations, interpretations and experiences of looking at photographs and discussing issues with family become, in turn, the basis for changing themselves.

Briefly summarized, looking at photographs and albums provides family members with the opportunity to reestablish contact with close relatives that are distant (or with distant relatives), to learn family history, to deal with unresolved issues (often the source of current anxiety and problems), and the opportunity to take the responsibility for their part in the operation of the family systems. Bowen family systems theory provides a framework to guide the formation of questions and hypotheses about individuals and relationships as expressed in the photographs.

The examples that follow show how the concepts of family systems theory can be operationalized and used in family therapy for the observation of photograph albums. As such, they are neither definitive nor exhaustive, but indicative of the manner in which the technique flows from the theory. Photographs can be read many times and in many ways to communicate the wealth of information they contain; the examples can be used to interpret and illustrate several different concepts simultaneously. The examples are provided to stimulate therapists to think creatively about how they may apply the concepts of family systems theory to the observation of relationship patterns in the family in the study of photographs and family photograph albums.

Triangles

Triangles deal with emotional closeness and distance between two individuals and the role of a third person (or issue/object) in that relationship. The patterns of interaction of the twosome in the relationship determines how anxiety is handled in the relationship. In triangles there are two insiders and one outsider. During periods of calm, the inside position is preferred. During periods of high tension and stress, the outside position is preferred, since the position is relatively free from the anxiety of the twosome. In times of low stress, the insiders are relatively close and the outsider feels isolated. "All family

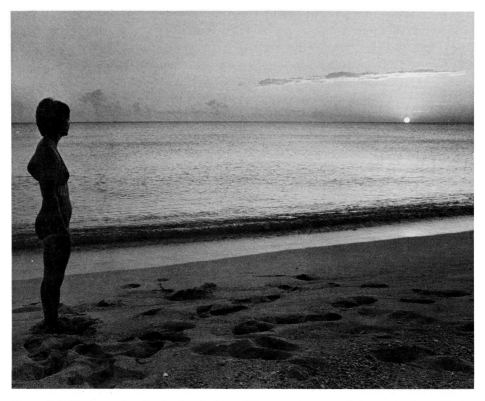

Figure 7-1. Horizon triangle: A triangle formed by two viewers and the sun in line with the horizon. A sculpture.   Photo by Michael Crane, 1974.

members have contributed equally to the process. Just as an individual cannot be understood outside of the context of their important relationships, no relationship can be understood out of the context of the way it interlocks with other family relationships. The calm or harmony in one relationship can be maintained by the conflict in another relationship" (Kerr, 1981, pp. 241-2).

The concept of triangles illuminates the innovative manner in which technique follows theory. When a twosome reviews photos, especially when direct talk about family issues is too tense, the photo album can serve as the third leg of a triangle. This creatively focuses the tension outside of the twosome and "onto" the photo album. Furthermore, it becomes easier to talk about pictures, even of the individuals involved, because while it is a picture of them, it is not them. Thus, each viewer can get enough distance and objectivity to observe and talk about self. Using the process of reviewing photographs with family members as a way of dealing with relationship issues, as well as renewing (distant or remote) relationships in the present, helps individuals to "detriangle" themselves from the intensity of the issues involved.

Another version of a triangle is that created when an individual looks at photograph albums for the purpose of reminiscing and thinking about previous memories and relationships. As expressed by one woman:

Sometimes when I get low in spirits and feeling badly . . . sort of wondering if life is worth living and all that . . . then I'll go and get the large box of old photos I have and pull them out. After I look at them, certain memories come back to me, memories that I think I've forgotten . . . looking at the pictures you wouldn't think it would have any direct connection with the pictures, but it evokes other memories . . . perhaps one person in the picture will remind me of something else . . . another memory. . . . The result is that the bad feelings go away and I'm in a good mood and hopeful again . . . no longer down in the dumps.

Triangles can also be observed in pictures by studying the spatial closeness, distance aspects of relationships as potentially mirroring the emotional. The accumulation of repeated images helps to differentiate between more temporary alliances and patterns and more characteristic relationship patterns. Some leads for questions and observations of pictures include:

Who are the people involved?
How are they grouped?
Who is touching/close to whom?
Is one person always in the center of the photograph?
Is one person always off to one side?
What position are the children in?
Is the oldest/middle/youngest always in the "favored" position between the parents?
Is your mother/father (in-law) hovering over you or your spouse?

The information from a single photograph might be overinterpreted since it might reflect only the mood of the moment. Hence pictures over a period of time have to be studied. In answering the above questions, it is important to attempt to differentiate temporary from characteristic patterns and look for flexibility and variety in patterns and groupings. Fixed patterns, someone always off alone, apart from the family, may be indicative of a close, overinvolved relationship between family members and an emotionally distant, isolated third member of a triangular pattern. In contrast, where these patterns of relationships may not be as apparent in the pictures, perhaps where there is more variety in the way the family poses and who stands next to whom changes frequently, the photographs reflect a family relationship pattern that is more adaptive. It is also important for the individual looking at the photographs with the family to ask enough questions about the observations to confirm or invalidate the developing hypotheses about the relationship patterns.

A successful woman executive examined photographs of her family taken when she was growing up. Particularly striking was a series depicting her parents, older brother and herself. In each, her mother held her, her brother stood close by, leaning toward them, while her father, dressed like "out of the bandbox" always in a three-piece suit with his hands in his pockets, stood physically isolated from the family (Fig. 7-2). Tears came to her eyes as she discussed the emotional distance between her father and herself and the impossibility she felt of ever being able to get close to him or discuss important issues affecting her life with him. The same triangle pattern of distance with her husband and overinvolvement with her young daughter exists. Therapeutical-

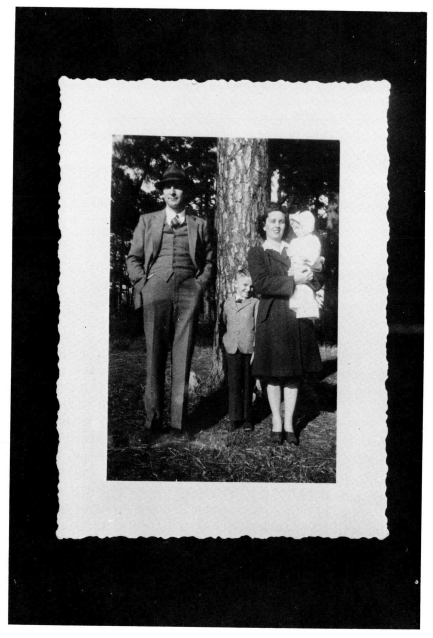

Figure 7-2.

ly, one of the tasks is to help her work on the relationship with her father and, as that distance is reduced, the changes can be translated into changes in her marital relationship.

Differentiation of Self

The concept of the differentiation of self attempts to conceptualize all human functioning on a continuum called the scale of differentiation. It defines how people are different with regard to managing issues of thinking versus feeling, individuality versus togetherness. People who live their lives in a feeling world, for whom the forces of togetherness (fusion) dominate, are at the lower end of the scale. With increasingly higher levels of differentiation, there is more of a balance between these opposing forces; and both systems become more separately defined and less reactive to each other. Thus, "the optimum mix or balance . . . permits the person to be a well defined individual in his/her own right as well as an effective team player" (Kerr, 1981, pp. 246-7). Family systems therapy is directed toward helping individuals differentiate a self in relationships in their family of origin, establish more open, personal and closer relationships, and thereby change their level of functioning.

The concept of a scale of differentiation has been mainly of theoretical, rather than empirical, importance. As such, it is difficult to operationalize visibly and directly in a photograph. Creative interpretations may permit the inference of this important concept.

An anonymous portrait of Sigmund Freud and his five sisters and a brother may serve as an example (Fig. 7-3). The caption published with it interprets his position and stance in the photograph as "the reserve and distance evident in the portrait are said to be consistent with Freud's later statements about his childhood" (Anonymous, 1979, p. 13). An alternative explanation suggests that Freud was less involved in the family togetherness and consequently able to achieve a more optimal level of differentiation, a level of well-defined individual functioning that would enable him to conceptualize about psychological development in a way that had not been done before him.

The lack of a differentiated relationship between a mother and professionally successful adult son was reflected in a series of photographs of the family. The man often faced his mother with a sad and longing look in his eyes. In one photograph he was actually on one knee, a seeming supplicant, his hand holding his mother's hand, with his mother in the center of the photograph and his whole extended family, including his new (and third) wife surrounding them. Emotional fusion was an obvious inference. This was supported by his current wife's statements that he was still very dependent on his mother, wanted desperately to please her and to prove to her that he was a "good boy" (Fig. 7-4).

At this time one can only speculate as to whether spaces between family members reflect distancing maneuvers or a family system that permits differentiation of its members. It may depend, also, on the point of view of the family member looking at and interpreting the pictures.

In the process of differentiating a self a person has to work on relationships with members of the family of origin. An interesting aspect of this process may be reflected in their efforts at photographing their family. Bowen emphasizes the difficulties that may be involved in working on a relationship with

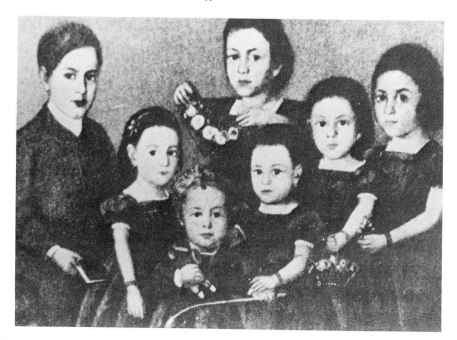

Figure 7-3. An anonymous portrait of Sigmund Freud (upper left) and his five sisters and brother. The reserve and distance evident in the portrait are said to be consistent with Freud's later statements about his childhood. Reprinted by permission of Mary Evans Picture Library.

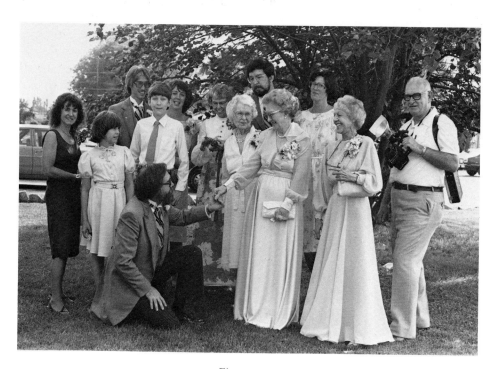

Figure 7-4.

Photo by Alan D. Entin

one's father and mother. Ralph Hattersley's experience with family photographs is similar. Although millions of photographs are taken each year of parents, he suggests that these snapshots are superficial since the individuals "neither see what they are photographing nor think about it" (1976, p. 237). In his book *Discover Your SELF Through Photography,* he describes his experiences as a teacher of photography when he told his students to photograph their parents. He stressed that "you must look at them as human beings with feelings, not just as objects to point your camera at . . . *Think* about your parents while you are photographing. *Think* about them as finite human beings, who have the same needs and emotions as you do. . . . (The directions were) the verbal equivalent to a hand grenade. In effect, I was asking each student to pick up a grenade, pull the firing pin, then clutch it to his breast" (pp. 237-8). The results were "disastrous" and, for some, the experience "(s)o painful . . . (that) they could not stand to use a camera again. Most were immobilized for a month or two. Some for years. A few even left photography altogether" (p. 237).

This vivid account underscores the importance of working on relationships with one's own family; the relationship will be reflected in the photos. All photographs take place in a context; the context is the social relationship between the photographer and the subject (Entin, 1980).

What do "favorite" photographs reveal about individuals' views of themselves, their parents and the emotional process operating in their family at the time of the picture? Although not yet explored, would "hated" photographs be equally revealing? How do the visual images compare with the stories, myths and legends that are recalled verbally? Are the minislices of family life captured real or idealized versions of the family? The pictures are most valuably interpreted by those who are in the photographs, and therefore only vulnerable to their projective inferences.

It is interesting to speculate as to how a less differentiated, or emotionally fused, family might assemble a photo album as compared with a more differentiated, less togetherness-oriented, family. It appears that a less differentiated family, perhaps vulnerable under stress to more anxiety, may assemble an album with a unitary point of view. This thematic expression is highlighted in "The Perfect Family (Album)" assembled by a woman who was terminally ill as a present to her young daughter (Entin, 1982). It showed the aspects of the family and the characteristics the mother perceived as important. There were no photos of the mother and daughter, a striking example of the distance and lack of relationship between them.

A twenty-one-year-old client was encouraged to review the photos taken when she was a young girl. Rather than follow through at home, she decided to look at them during the next therapy session. There were several dramatic features. This was not an album about her. Instead, she brought in an album of her younger twin brothers, assuming most of her pictures were in relation to them. Continuing the drama was her differential relationship to the twins. In virtually every picture of her and the boys, she was either touching or standing closest to the same brother! And, when one was photographed individually, it was usually the other brother, seldom the one she said was emotionally closer to her. When she asked her father about these coincidences, he vigorously denied the obvious visual evidence. Furthermore, even in several studio portraits of all three children, the girl was always next to the same brother as in the informal snapshots. Is this evidence of fused relationships operating?

Sibling Position

Since a family relationship begins with two people, the husband and wife, it is interesting to observe what happens when a third person, the first child, is born. How the relationship between the spouses changes with the birth of the first child can also be interpreted as understanding the triangles in the family.

> How do the photographs taken before the child was born compare with the ones snapped after the child is born?
> Who is more emotionally involved or responsible for the caretaking of the child?
> Is the mother always holding the child? The father? One of the grandparents?
> Do the people look relaxed with the child or is there obvious discomfort and tension in their expressions and poses?
> Do the expressions reflect joy or resentment?
> Would there be a difference in the responses to a boy or girl?
> Do these patterns change over time?

When the next child is born, the three-person system changes to a four-person system. Previously established relationships are altered.

> What happens when the second child is born?
> Is there a different response to the first born and second born?
> Does the first child remain in the center of the picture or does the new baby take center stage?
> What happens when other children are born into the family?
> Do the relationships change?
> In what ways?
> Are the changes consistent over time?
> Is there a difference between how boys and girls are portrayed?

Is one child photographed more than the others? Typically first-born children are photographed more than later-born children, and most photographs are taken while the children are relatively young and changing. However, if a second-born child is photographed significantly more than the first-born, for example, hypotheses can be raised regarding the child's meeting the expectations of the family with regard to such issues as its sex or attractiveness, or because of some family secret such as illegitimacy, handicap or disfigurement. When family members become adamant about trying to keep the number of photographs of the first and second child the same, issues such as equality and favoritism are also raised (Entin, 1982).

Emotional Cutoff

The concept of emotional cutoff describes one way people deal with unresolved togetherness (fusion) in their family of origin. This can typically be done through emotional cutting off or physical distance from the family, and/or withdrawal or avoidance of emotionally charged issues while with the family. This concept is important as "a cornerstone of family psychotherapy based on this version of family systems theory" (Kerr, 1981, p. 250). Its significance is in the role the "existence of or reestablishment of viable emotional contact between three or more generations of a family can be (as) an important symptom-reducing influence . . . it is not just a simple matter of going home for a visit. The intensity of the emotional forces that created the cutoff must be understood and respected" (Kerr, 1981, p. 250).

In looking at albums it is, then, also extremely important to take into account the people who are not in the picture, in addition to those who are photographed. What does a person's absence mean? During adolescence, individuals attempt to seek their own individuality and may deal with the family togetherness by cutting off from parents. This may occur in varying degrees of intensity ranging from long hair and blue jeans, emotional turmoil, acting-out behavior via emotional cutoffs from the family, or running away from home. The photo albums may provide clues as to the ways the relationship problems were dealt with in the family. Typically, during periods of family stress, conflict or crisis, there is a sharp decrease in the number of pictures taken. Obvious gaps may reveal times of family crisis, or the absence of an expected or significant figure may be attributable to an illness, hospitalization or emotional cutoff, and an inference may be made about the operation of the family emotional process. These assumptions, however, should be validated through discussions with family members. If there are many pictures of a particular child and then suddenly photos of that child are conspicuous by their absence, this could be indicative of a cutoff. Did a change in weight, dramatically graphic in photographs, reflect other changes in the family? Perhaps the "camera shy" child also reflects such emotional upsets. A vivid portrayal of a cutoff is a photograph where an individual is "cutoff" (cut out) of the picture (Fig. 7-5). This demonstrates that cutoffs do not "solve" problems because the individual "cut off" is still there (present by the absence) and, therefore, the cutoff continues to exist until the issues are resolved.

In a similar manner the family life cycle may be studied through the photo album. What is chosen to be photographed, recorded and documented for the album reflects the ideals, traditions and values of the family. Significant information is provided by looking at nodal events, ceremonies and rites of passage over time, noting changes in who is present and who is absent. This provides evidence of possible emotional cutoffs, as well as attempts to reestablish contacts, in families. "(W)ho appears at which event" is "not accidental" according

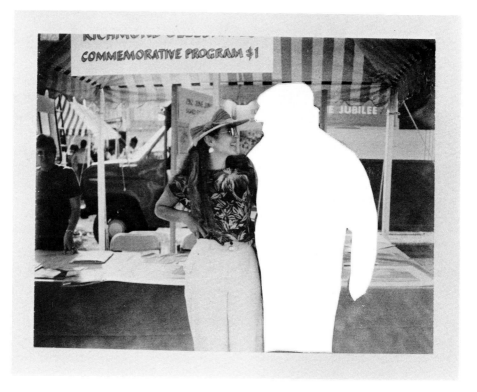

Figure 7-5.

Photo by Alan D. Entin

to Friedman (1980, p. 432) in a discussion of the way families deal with ceremonies relating to transitions and rites of passage. These occasions provide individuals with the opportunity to reenter the family and reestablish contacts with distant relatives or close relatives who are distant for the purpose of dealing with the issues which may have contributed to the cutoff.

In another family there was an abundance of pictures of children alone, with each other, and with the father. Questioning revealed that the parents were divorced, the mother had primary custody and the father occasional visitation rights. The father's overreaction to feeling isolated and cut off from the children was reflected in the abundance of pictures, as if to deny the reality of his absence from the family.

THE FAMILY PHOTO ALBUM AS ICON

To recapitulate, photographs and family albums communicate information about individuals and relationship patterns in the family. Emphasis in my clinical work is placed on family systems theory as an organizing framework to help individuals understand the part each family member plays in the operation of the relationship system. Such information then enables the individual to do something about one's part in the system: to change. When one is able to change, one can effect changes in other parts of the system. The use of family albums is a technique to assist in the understanding of the family system, reestablish contact with family members, and deal with unresolved issues to change one's self. The interpretation and analysis of photographs, per se, is not the focus of my clinical use of photographs in family psychotherapy. I usually do not sit down with individuals to look at their pictures or albums. Instead, they are encouraged to do this with their parents, outside the therapy sessions, although individuals may decide to bring their albums to a therapy session.

The focus of this chapter has been on some of the manifold ways that the concept of Bowen family systems theory may be manifest or inferred in photographs and family albums. The concepts of triangles is particularly helpful to show the innovations which can follow from this theory. In the field of photography and psychotherapy, this paper is the latest in a series of efforts to develop the application of Bowen family systems theory. By learning how to "read" photographs using the concepts of family systems theory, it then becomes possible to observe and interpret albums more sensitively to understand better one's own personal and family history. They visually articulate the meaning of the relationships of the family while serving as landmarks for a history of continuity and change within the multigenerational family portrait. Their significance over and above the images renders the family photo album as icon.

> The picture of the mind revives again:
> While here I stand, not only with the sense of present pleasure, but with pleasing
> thoughts that in this moment there is life and food for future years.
>
> William Wordsworth
> 1770-1850

REFERENCES

Anonymous, Photo Psychology. *Innovations,* American Institutes for Research, Palo Alto, Cal., Winter 1979, *Vol. 6, No. 3,* p. 13.

Barrow, T.F. Learning from the past. In J. Alinder, (Ed.), *Nine critics/Nine photographers.* Carmel, California: The Friends of Photography, 1980, p. 32-36.

Bowen, M. Family and family group therapy. In H. Kaplan and B. Sadock (Eds.), *Comprehensive group psychotherapy.* Baltimore: Williams and Wilkins, 1971.

Bowen, M. Toward the differentiation of a self in one's own family. In J. Framo (Ed.), *Family interaction — A dialogue between family researchers and family therapists.* New York: Springer Publishing Co., 1972.

Bowen, M. Theory in the practice of pyschotherapy. In P. Guerin (Ed.). *Family therapy: Theory and practice.* New York: Gardner, 1976.

Bowen, M. *Family therapy in clinical practice.* New York: Aronson, 1978.

Crane, M. Horizon Triangle/A Sculpture. Photograph in *Tri Quarterly 32,* Winter, 1975.

De Lappa, W. Regeneration: Images and Icons. *Photo America* Announcement, 1981.

Entin, A.D. The Genogram: A Multigenerational Family Portrait. Paper presented at the American Psychological Association, August 29, 1978.

Entin, A.D. Photo Therapy: Family Albums and Multigenerational Portraits. *Camera Lucida,* 1980, *Vol. 2, No. 2,* 39-51.

Entin, A.D. The Use of Photographs and Family Albums in Family Therapy. In A. Gurman (Ed.), *Questions and answers in the practice of family psychotherapy.* New York: Brunner/Mazel, 1981.

Entin, A.D. Family Icons: Photographs in Family Psychotherapy, In L. Abt, and I. Stuart (Eds.), *The newer therapies: A sourcebook.* New York: Van Nostrand, 1982, 207-227.

Entin, E.S. Personal Communication, Oct, 21, 1981.

Fenjves, P.F. Understanding family may be a snap. *Chicago Sun Times,* Nov. 20, 1981, p. 16-17.

Friedman, E.H. Systems and Ceremonies: A Family View of Rites of Passage. In E. Carter and M. McGoldrick (Eds.), *The family life cycle.* New York: Gardner Press, 1980.

Hattersley, R. *Discover your SELF through photography.* Dobbs Ferry, New York: Morgan & Morgan, 1976.

Kerr, M.E. Family Systems Theory and Therapy. In A. Gurman and D. Kniskern (Eds.), *Handbook of family therapy.* New York: Brunner/Mazel, 1981.

Wordsworth, W. Lines Composed a Few Miles Above Tintern Abbey. In A.J.M. Smith (Ed.), *Seven centuries of verse.* New York: Charles Scribner's Sons, 1947, p. 307.

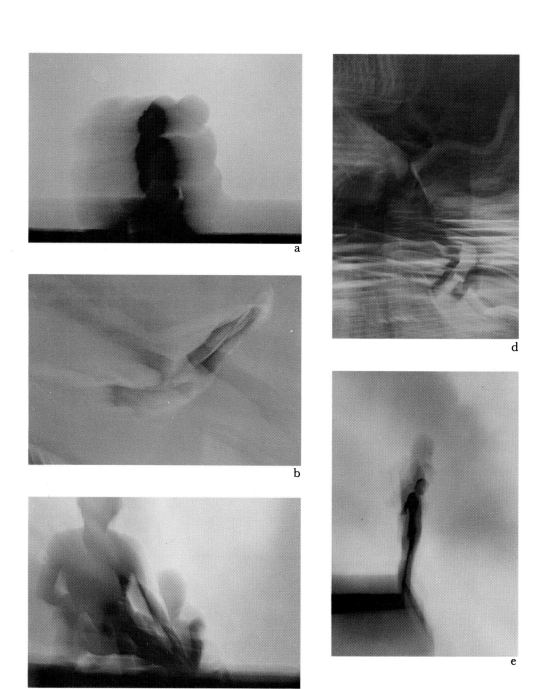

a

b

c

d

e

Plate 1

Chapter 8

The Photograph as a Catalyst in Psychotherapy

Joel Walker

INTRODUCTION

THE purpose of this paper is to describe the utility and efficacy of a new technique to facilitate the psychotherapeutic process. This approach involves a new application of projective techniques. I am using photographic images for the primary purpose of therapeutics in contrast to an emphasis on diagnostic usage. The concept of phototherapy is not new as the use of photographs in a psychiatric setting was first used by Dr. Hugh Diamond in 1856. He recorded the physiological appearance of various types of mental illness on admission and discharge and the treatment of the mentally ill through the presentation of an accurate self-image.

I will first discuss the images that I use in my practice and then give an historical perspective of the process that I have gone through in developing these approaches. Finally, I will integrate these approaches within the framework of some of the major issues in psychotherapy demonstrated by some case histories.

THE IMAGES

Projectives such as the Rorschach and TAT were designed as tests for the purpose of assessment. Unlike the Rorschach images, which are totally unreal, and the TAT images, which are very real, my photographic pictures are purposely ambiguous and abstract but have a semblance of reality. The images themselves, though basically abstract, are representational enough to imply either singular thoughts or actions, or relationships between individuals. They are ambiguous images of suffused color and shadowy form that attempt to leave everything to the imagination. The images allow the viewer to project onto them their own gestalt, the way they perceive the world at a given moment in time. If you want someone to free-associate and to fantasize, you want to give them the widest range possible. There are no titles on these pictures so as not to

135

give the viewers any preconceived ideas. Some are slightly more abstract, some less, and that is to purposefully give a range so that people can relate to different ones, as some people are more comfortable with more abstract images than others. Clearly, the more abstract the image, the greater the opportunity to project. They are unstructured which by design permits interpretation. The patient can project upon the photograph his way of seeing life, its meaning, significances, patterns, relationships, and especially feelings. The images are confronting — there is no place to run in the photograph. The patient either deals with the image or not. Most of the prints are monochromatic giving the viewer few clues with which to work.

With the abstract images, people quickly begin to structure them in the way they tend to deal with their own world. They take these unstructured stimuli and put them together in the way they live in the outside world or their inner world. How one copes and how one relates is reflected in this process. I found it very economical in that it could quickly cut through resistance and define major conflict areas.

HISTORICAL PERSPECTIVE

When I first opened my office, I realized that I would be spending many hours a day there so I wanted to make it as comfortable as possible. I started to put up pictures, photographs which I had taken. Understandably, when patients come to a psychiatrist's office, many feel quite apprehensive. They wonder what will happen to them inside these four walls. They question whether something will be taken from them and what they will become. I found that what many of them would do would be to comment about the images that were up on the walls, things which were seemingly outside of themselves. In fact, what they were revealing was what they were feeling at that moment.

There are several things that I am implicitly saying to my patients by putting up my own photographs in the office; that I have a right to enjoy, to have a life outside of my practice, and to be multifaceted — many patients cannot imagine their psychiatrist having a life outside of the office walls. These implicit messages act as vicarious modelling for handling their own life. The photographs on the walls are subtle statements that they, the patients, are potentially free.

The next historical development occurred as I decided to use the images in a directive manner as well as in the spontaneous, quiet-initiated approach. This latter was a nondirective technique. I became aware that if I did not become directive, I would be colluding with my patients in the knowledge that they really had a lot of feelings about the fact that their psychiatrist was a photographer too, and a funny artist at that. They would wonder "How come he always likes fuzzy things? — Doesn't he like people?" How did he manage to become a psychiatrist and a photographer too? There could be lots of feelings of jealousy and competitiveness, and if I didn't deal with these feelings, they could hinder the therapeutic process. In terms of respecting my patients and the therapeutic relationship, I felt I had a responsibility to become directive. By that I mean I had to make a clinical decision to actually initiate discussion.

My primary purpose in both the directive and nondirective approaches is to use the patient's responses to the photographs in order to achieve therapeutic goals. Each of the responses is best interpreted in the context of the whole situation, being aware of the history and what is going on in therapy over time. People respond differently depending upon their own mental set and their individual life situation and background. If in an ambiguous image a patient feels that he sees a ten-foot spider, of course it raises my index of suspicion, but the response must be seen in context. For example, often gifted people respond with what appear to be pathological responses. Isolated responses often mean nothing in themselves. What is important is what follows from the response. It is the dialogue and thematic content that is pursued that is essential. It is how they knit the response into the fabric of their lives that is important. The context is essential; for example, a creative artist, schizophrenic and a child may all perceive the same thing.

The initial response gives me additional cues of where to go from here. It acts as a cuing mechanism. For example, a sexual response may lead to an opportunity to talk about the patient's fears or inadequacy. It may be that the response was triggered off by something deeply rooted in the past or perhaps merely the anticipation of a date that would be occurring the next day. My follow-up comments may be based on past responses of the patient or my interpretation of underlying dynamics. Some photographs elicit certain responses more consistently than others. General themes given by my patients otherwise well defended include the following: loneliness, low self-esteem, problems with intimacy, rage, fear of losing control, dependence-independence conflict, anger and depression. These reflect the kinds of difficulties they have or experience. The images are really the beginning of dialogue. I found that they were more helpful in terms of breaking through resistance, mobilizing affect, and useful in terms of transference.

The next historical development involved my participation in photographic exhibits. Due to the nature of my work with patients in a clinical setting using photographs as an adjunct in therapy, I felt that it was important to have a larger data base from which I could become aware of normative responses — the range of responses, the typical and atypical ones, and the predominant thematic content. Therefore, when I had a photographic exhibit, I chose to make it a participatory experience. The way people look at photographs reflects the way they feel. It is these feelings that influence the way an image is perceived. These ideas are the basis of an exhibition of my photographs called "See And Tell." Because of my interest in how people respond to photographs in the office, I wondered how would the general population respond. Not only did I think this might be helpful in terms of a comparison between my patient population and a general population, I thought it would be an enjoyable learning experience for the gallery goer. I entitled my exhibits "See And Tell" and showed the images in New York, Toronto and Mexico City (see *Time* magazine article entitled "See And Tell": Color Phototherapy, August 17/81, pp. 34-35).

The exhibition was unique in that it involved audience participation. The viewers were invited to write down their individual responses, specifically their feelings and fantasies elicited by the ten images. Beneath each photograph were two boxes: one labeled "Take It," containing cards labeled "Tell," and another labeled "Leave It." where viewers deposited their responses. The viewers were free to compare their responses to those of other people. There were no right or wrong answers. Because I wanted the show to be open-ended and fun, I allowed the responses to remain anonymous so that the experience would be as nonthreatening as possible. This informal survey, therefore, does not claim to be scientific in any sense, as my primary purpose was to explore areas for further development. Generally, the exhibit was an opportunity for people to become aware of their own feelings and compare their perceptions with those of others. I was hoping that the public would become aware that there are many ways to perceive abstract art and that it is O.K. to feel whatever you are feeling. The underlying method of the exhibits was that everyone's perceptions and feelings are worthwhile, and I found that the responses that people wrote down really began to tell a lot about them. These normative responses in the general population gave me some idea of the typical and atypical responses that I might expect.

Over the three weeks I collected approximately 4,000 responses and personally interviewed many individuals who passed through the exhibit. People seemed to be committed to the show, spending from 15 minutes to one hour experiencing the images. A number of people came back several times, perceiving the images differently on subsequent visits. As a psychiatrist, I am interested in both intra- and interpersonal dynamics. One woman came in and responded to four photographs, then stopped. When I observed the closure, I asked her why she had stopped. She said, "I became aware of the fact that I was really talking about myself. And I wasn't ready to deal with that." Another person came in with his father and said, "I rarely do things together with my dad. This gives us a chance to talk about some of the things we are feeling." This experience with the exhibits was the prelude to my use of the cards in my practice. A variation of this experience in a clinical setting was utilized and is illustrated in the final case history.

Basically there are two categories of techniques, the nondirective and the directive.

The nondirective is a spontaneous response by the patient to a photograph. This may occur at any time in the course of therapy. By allowing this spontaneity, I am implicitly saying that comments are permissible and desirable and that patients have the right to feel and express feelings.

The directive approach is where I make a clinical decision to inquire about the photograph. This may involve a random selection of two or three photographs in an informal fashion, or more formally structured by requesting that the patient respond to all ten images in written form. The techniques are different, but the resultant process is the same, to activate dialogue around the relevant theme. Thus, the photograph acts as a catalyst through which the dialogue transpires and awareness is encouraged.

CASE ILLUSTRATIONS

The last section of this chapter will focus upon the utility and efficacy of these approaches within the framework of some of the major issues in psychotherapy demonstrated by case history.

The primary focus of this section will be on the directive approach; however, first I will give one example of the spontaneous nondirective approach and then pursue the directive approach in more depth. This first case history illustrates the emergence of transferential phenomena in dynamic psychotherapy through the presence or absence of an image. (see Plate 1a).

Case #1

Susan is a twenty-seven-year-old divorced female who works in marketing and who lives with a childhood friend who is in the same marital situation as she. Susan is an only child of Spanish heritage. She was referred because of anxiety, confusion and feelings of guilt. Her major problems lay in the areas of her sexual identity, intimacy and a poor sense of self.

DIALOGUE: Susan walks into my office, sits down, looks around and after a long pause asks me, "Where are the pictures?" I say, "What did you imagine happened to them?" Susan replied, "Had the pictures offended someone?" "Did you personally not want them up?" pause, she continued, "I don't want to talk about it." I said, "I think it's important to try and talk about it." She then said, "Who were the photos of?" "Are the photos of you and your wife undressed?" "Do you want to take them down because everyone is looking at them?" I replied, "The photos are of a silver medalist from the Commonwealth Games and his wife dressed." "How would you feel if it was me in the photos undressed?" I asked. She replied, "A side of you I have never seen before. Do you actually live outside of this office?" Then, staring at the table Susan paused. I said, "What are you thinking right now?" She replied, "Thinking, I don't see you as a person, you're not a friend — it's strange; it makes me anxious — who are you?" I said, "What comes to mind?" and Susan replied, "I can't imagine you anywhere else but in this room . . . one little room . . . I don't see a person. I don't understand this — how can I be telling you all these things — this isn't a relationship" . . . This is a cause of a great sense of anxiety. "I feel indignant — How dare you have this life outside of my problems. I feel possessive — Get those damn things off the wall. Why are you asking me so much about this photo?" I answered, "Because it's a part of me that was in this room and you have a lot of feelings about it." Susan said, "You deliberately took them off. You just wanted to see what I was going to say." Long pause . . . I asked, "What are you feeling right now?" She replied, "How awful it is to be alone."

PROCESS: Susan was able to express her feelings about me which is essential to the therapeutic process. Because she views most relationships with men as she viewed her relationship with her father, and ex-husband; example lacking in intimacy, affection and trust, she went on to project those same characteristics onto me. The absence of the photographs, allowed Susan to express feelings about me which she had not to date otherwise expressed. Just as she experienced a childhood and early womanhood lacking in intimacy and trust, it soon became apparent to both of us that Susan expected the same kind of treatment from me. This is not to suggest that this issue of transference would not have come out in subsequent sessions, however, the photographs or absence of photographs in this case encouraged an earlier exploration than might have otherwise been anticipated.

This technique can reduce the patient's anxieties and the photograph relates to something seemingly external to themselves. I say "seemingly" because often it is difficult to divorce one's self from one's feelings because one's own experiences influence the way we perceive the world. It is economical as well for it brings up feelings that may not be apparent due to a projective nature. It increases available data and may reduce resistance to therapy.

The next case history illustrates how one photograph became invaluable in breaking through resistance.

Case #2

John was a married man in his early thirties who was trying to get his degree in optometry. He was referred to me because he thought he was having a heart attack and dying and had been to one cardiologist after another, none of whom could find anything wrong with him. He had a burning pain in his chest and he seemed to be getting it all the time.

PROCESS: Any time a psychological interpretation was made, it was met with resistance and he'd go running off to see his cardiologist again. As this cycle kept recurring, I began to feel more and more frustrated. I felt it was a psychosomatic problem and not his heart. Enough cardiologists had seen John, and he looked pretty healthy to me. After making a clinical decision to ask him to respond to some of the images, I came to one image and there was suddenly a tremendous amount of fury and rage that was unleashed. He literally went into a rage and then his feelings about himself in relation to his father came pouring out. Despite exploring this issue in previous sessions, the intensity of his feelings had never become apparent to either one of us. The image really triggered this awareness. As he began to deal with his own rage and anger, the pains began to subside and eventually left him. The image became an economical means to cut through the resistance to therapy.

The next case history involves working through conflict.

Case #3

Mary is a depressed lady in her mid-fifties who is very religious and moral. She has been a foster mother for thirty different babies at various times in her life. She and her husband have two of their own daughters who are presently living on the periphery of society and having children out of wedlock. Her depression was primarily focused upon her two daughters.

PROCESS: Whenever we explored the relationship between Mary and her daughters, her ambivalence was always apparent. She loved them as daughters but didn't really like them as people. She couldn't accept what they had become or the demands she felt they had imposed on her. One of them was going to be having a baby out of wedlock and this made her terribly upset. The same daughter had a previous pregnancy which terminated in a stillborn birth, and Mary was fearful that the present pregnancy would end the same way. At this point, I made a clinical decision to ask her to respond to one of the images hanging on the wall. Her back was towards it but she turned around and trembling began to describe moving arms and some semblance of legs but no body — it reminded her of a fetus. She left the session and came back the next time saying, "I thought you were supposed to help me. I have had nothing but nightmares since I left here. I am really upset and I can't get that bloody image out of my head. That's all I ever see. I don't want to see that picture." Then, she turned her back to the picture. As I encouraged her to talk about her feelings, she related how she had been called right to the delivery room the previous time and how traumatic the whole birthing process had been. The image acted as a vehicle to epitomize the unconscious conflict and her intense fear about her repressed concerns involving the whole birthing process. It was interesting that once the child was born in a normal delivery she came to the session several weeks later and was able to find the entire fetus in a different location in the image. Whereas in her previous projection she could only perceive disintegration, there was now a completion, a whole. The visual image of the dismembered fetus had remained with her, she was confronted by it and this confrontation had forced her to unleash the repressed fear.

In the next two examples, the approach is more formalized, structured and extensive in contrast to prior approaches. Here the patient was asked to respond in a written form to the ten images as employed in the photographic exhibit. The following case is illustrative of the use of the photograph and its role in formulation.

Case #4

Michael is a divorced salesman in his early thirties who is bright, well-dressed and involved in a number of superficial relationships. He was very manipulative, cold and distant. He had many of the characteristics of a psychopath. An interesting feature of this case was that he owed me money. There is recognition in Michael's mind that there is a discrepancy between the way he perceives himself and the way others would perceive him.

PROCESS: I worked with him for about six months, during which time he was quite intellectual. He couldn't talk about his past and he tended to block his early experiences under ten years of age. It was very difficult to elicit any feelings from Michael. I decided to deal with the money situation as it was directly related to me and concrete. I said to him, "What's your fantasy? Do you think that because I'm a psychiatrist that I make a lot of money and I don't need the earth? I get the feeling that you don't ever intend to pay me." He replied, "If you feel that way maybe I should get the money." I said, "What do you mean if I feel that way? If somebody said that to me, I would feel anxious and angry. I would think he's probably right for putting me on the spot. How are you feeling?" Michael replied, "Nothing, I don't feel anything but I understand the position you're in." At this point, I decided to ask Michael to respond to all ten images, almost as a last resort to try to tap whether in fact he had any feelings at all.

The following are several examples of Michael's responses. I asked him to write down his thoughts, feelings and fantasies, particularly his feelings, about the following images.

FIGURE 8-1: "Aerial shots of a large island with small lakes and a heavy wooded area."

PLATE 1b: "It is a woman diving into water with nylons on and a blue top or she is flying on a trapeze swing."

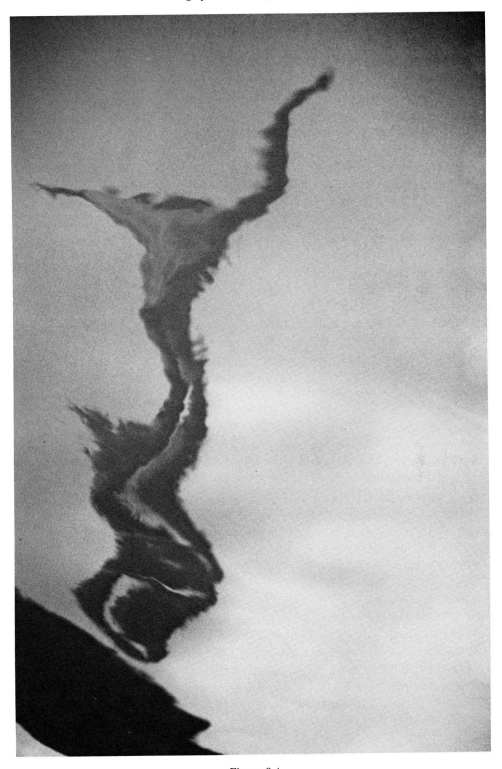

Figure 8-1.

PLATE 1c: "This is a mother preparing food, perhaps baking. Father is at the table behind her reading a paper and keeping her company."

Michael's responses had an empty quality to them. There was no sense of himself and he took no risks. After he had written down his responses, I asked him to read them over and verbally respond to what he wrote down. I said to him, "Pretend that these written responses are someone else's and describe what you would say about the way that person responded." He just restated what he had written. That was all he could make out of it, so I handed him a group of anonymous responses by some other patients. Some people write down responses which have a poverty of affect, as did Michael's responses. Others are capable of responding with feeling but there is an objective tone to the ownership of these feelings. And still others, respond with feeling and are subjective about the ownership of these feelings. When I handed the other responses to Michael, he grabbed his head and said, "Look — there is no way, no way that I could do any of that, I can't even relate to that. I didn't even think people could talk like that." While looking at the response cards, it made him aware of the fact that there were other possibilities, that he in fact was extremely devoid of feeling. He was like a child wanting to learn again. In prior sessions, I had seen him as a psychopath, but this man was not a psychopath. He was so empty and deprived of any feelings or experience. We began, then, to delve into his background when he was a child. The realization was that there were no emotions, warmth or support in his past. My own counter-transference had got in the way of my empathy. The fact that I saw him as a psychopath did not allow me to deal with him effectively. Through the use of the photographs, I reformulated this case, no longer perceiving Michael in this way. This affected the counter-transference which in turn improved the rapport between us.

The utility of the above approach was its facilitation of a reformulation. My formulation was incomplete in the way that I had been dealing with Michael. The utility for him is the awareness it developed in him that there are potentially other ways of responding and that in the process of learning new ways, he must take risks.

The written responses allowed two projections to occur. Firstly, the patient had to project visually onto the image and secondly, this projection had to be translated into words; a black and white statement of the first projection became a valid tool whereby he could objectively see that there was something lacking in his own responses. If I had shown him other written responses in contrast to his own verbal statements, it would likely not have made the same impact.

The final case history exemplifies the process I have gone through in developing the use of photographs in my practice. This is one of the longest cases I have worked with and in fact I am continuing to work with him at this point in time. The psychotherapeutic issue which will be emphasized will be the one of affect. The following thumbnail sketch is a description of Steve when he first came into therapy.

Case #5

Steve is a man in his early forties who is married with two children. He has a Ph.D. in mineralogy and does consultation work in his field. Steve was referred during a depressive episode. The major underlying affect was anxiety. He was constantly running from exploring himself. As my photos are abstract and interpretive their projective use allowed this patient to identify and feel with something external to himself. This was less threatening for him than exploring something directly related to himself and therefore reduced his anxiety to evoking feelings rather than to deny and/or intellectualize his feelings. He was extremely analytical, conceptual and very bright.

DIALOGUE: I asked, "What feelings, fantasies or thoughts does this image (Plate 1d) evoke in you?" There was a prolonged silence, then Steve responded without hesitancy. "It looks like a reflection on a surface — metallic — irregular — meshwork. It reminds me of shapes seen in French caves — the crude outline — it has an analytic feeling to it."

At this point I thought that the response was indicative of how Steve sees his world. It is conspicuous by the absence of affective content, it is an intellectual analysis. Then, I said, "It's interesting that while I asked you what you felt when you looked at the image, I had the feeling that I was hearing you describe one of your rock specimens." He answered, "I guess I never really realized how difficult it is for me to talk about what I feel inside."

PROCESS: The dialogue around the photos continued over several sessions and finally focusing on himself he was able to respond with ease. Then he could deal with himself without the medium of photography. His way of coping in all situations was to approach them as a problem-to-be-solved. He had one great wrench which he used to deal with all situations. Feelings were foreign. In subsequent sessions, Steve learned to value himself and to know who he was, which allowed him to stop trying to prove his worth through his intelligence. Once he knew who he was, he began expressing his feelings. Steve's response helped confirm what I had surmised but most importantly it allowed him to recognize his difficulty.

About a year after the previous dialogue occurred, I asked Steve to respond to the ten images. I told him that I was interested in doing this from the point of view of progression.

PLATE 1a: "It's a vortex in the atmosphere. He sees it from the side sucking up the earth from below. It's not cold, but it's an inanimate feeling, transitory, recognizable, but no definite form. It's an intangible feeling."

PLATE 1e: "The last second before commitment. A figure about to dive. It is a feeling of being prepared. He is resigned to carry out the act. It's peaceful."

FIGURE 8-1: "A distortion of worn images by reflection. A feeling of confusion. A river seen through the clouds. The discovery of something known. Anxious to see beneath the featureless clouds. It is a feeling of height and searching."

Part of me got excited initially. I thought here he is using some feeling words. Steve has really moved a great deal. In fact he had; he was able to now use feelings. Then I began to look at it longer and felt that something was missing, and I showed his written responses to him. He looked at them for a long time and he said, "You know I don't really feel those things. It really is out there and it is much like watching something, being the observer and not being involved, being able to identify what the feelings ought to be but in fact not really feeling them at all." There was no ownership of feelings, he was a spectator.

Then he came up with a great idea because I showed him how other people had responded. There had been one girl in particular who I had seen the session before who was writing down "I don't like this image, I feel scared, it makes me nervous." He looked at it and he said, "You know I would like to try something in a couple of weeks. I would like to see if I could write the word 'I' in front of whatever I go to put down." We went through all the images again.

PLATE 1a: He said, "I feel cold about this photograph, there is no human contact." That's all he put down.

PLATE 1e: "I feel free."

FIGURE 8-1: "I would rather not look at this photograph. It is depressing, ugly and ominous, there is no warmth to it."

So, in fact, by his starting to use the word "I," he said that he began to get a different feeling about it. He said, "It's a lot easier than I thought it was going to be and that you know it's okay. I don't always have to deal with the world in one way. I don't always have to see it as a problem to be solved. I can in fact talk about what I feel and that's okay and feelings may even be more important than having to analyze everything."

This exercise acted as an evaluatory vehicle for both Steve and myself. He could actually see where he had come from and the progress he was making. He could also see his areas of weakness and the need for work in these areas, the example, ownership of feelings. One of the most exciting aspects for me was that this man who had previously been so rigid was able to become creative within this context and use the photographs in a way that could benefit him (example; using "I" to help him *own* feelings). The metamessage that I have always tried to give to my patients is that they are free, to choose, to decide, and to create.

CONCLUSION

This paper has focused upon the use of ambiguous photographs as a projective enabling the patient and therapist to more readily explore transferential feelings, penetrate resistance, work through conflicts, and mobilize affect. An historical overview was discussed and five case histories presented. In contrast to other projective techniques, the present discussion emphasized the therapeutic benefits in contrast to the diagnostic considerations. Its value as a catalyst in psychotherapy is further enhanced in its utility and efficacy in dealing with difficult cases as well as the not such difficult ones by acting as a tool which facilitates the psychotherapeutic process more readily.

Although two types of approaches were discussed, the nondirective client-initiated, spontaneous approach and the directive approach, the primary focus was on the latter technique. The directive approach was subdivided into the use of a select number of image(s) or the use of a series of ten images with the expectation that the patient respond in written form. This series-approach incorporated the use of other patients' anonymous responses as a sounding board in facilitating awareness and alternative response patterns.

Both techniques recognize that both patients and therapists have various perceptual styles. Some are perceived to be more analytical, verbal and rational, while others are more imaginative, visual and emotional to their approach in relating to the world. This addresses itself to the question of patient-therapist match which could lend itself to another article. Let me say at this point that by providing another tool for communication in the form of a visual vehicle, the match could be facilitated.

Some schools of thought believe that therapist self-disclosure and non-neutrality should be minimized. In this writer's use of phototherapy there is a conscious and deliberate exposure as the photos are a personal extension of the therapist. This disclosure gives further grist for the psychotherapeutic mill.

The catalytic use of photographs is an alternate strategy to explore the unconscious. With regard to the patients, it helps them verbalize, recognize feelings, fantasize, and often to realize an untapped storehouse of imagination and/or creative potential. It allows them to view themselves in a less defended way through the visual realm. As a society we place a high value on verbalization and we have learned how to defend ourselves intellectually. I believe that although feelings, thoughts and fantasies are expressed verbally in reaction to the photographs, that the visual impact overshadows the verbal defensive reppertoire. Finally, this method allows the patient to become more aware of his/her unique perception of the world.

"The photograph as a catalyst in psychotherapy" should not be viewed as a strategy in and of itself, but rather should be utilized as an integral part of the psychotherapeutic process. Just as my patients are learning and growing, I continue to experience the challenge of a new approach within my professional pursuits. Perhaps, the most exciting thing is that I am learning from my patients on a daily basis — it is not a one-way street.

REFERENCES

Medina, S. "See and Tell" Color Phototherapy. *Time Magazine,* August 17, 1981, pp. 34-35.
Walker, J. L. The photograph as a catalyst in psychotherapy. *Canadian Journal of Psychiatry,* October, 1982.

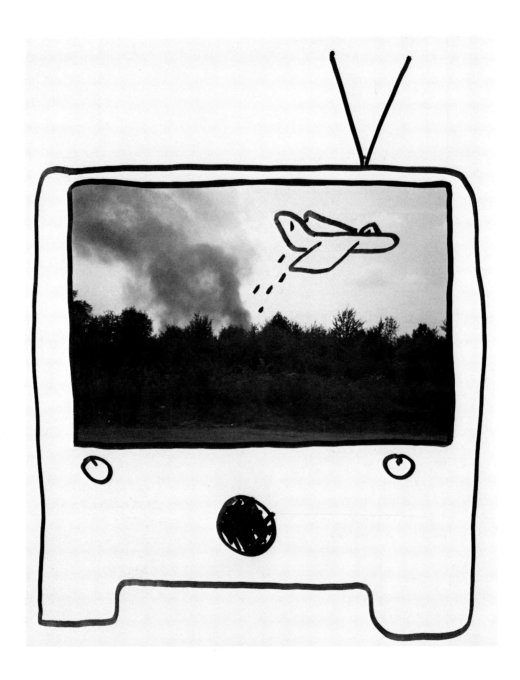

Photo by David A. Krauss

Chapter 9

Instant Phototherapy with Children and Adolescents

I NSTANT photography was first developed in 1948 by Dr. Edwin H. Land. This remarkable process enabled the photographer to view his finished print only minutes after the photo had been taken. The film was developed and printed automatically by chemicals that were located within the film cartridge and were activated by rollers which spread them over the film surface as the film was withdrawn from the camera.

Today this process has been refined. Instant photography is now easily available and quite simple to use. The process is quick and precise, and its results are so impressive that it is rapidly becoming a new art form for avante-garde photographers. As the reliability of the process improved and the cost of film and cameras lowered as a result of mass production, instant photography came within reach of psychotherapists who were looking for innovative techniques to reach patient populations difficult to motivate in traditional psychotherapy experiences. These early pioneers were especially struck by the impact this experience had upon autistic children, antisocial children, learning disabled children and acting-out adolescents, see e.g. Gee, 1976, Wolf, 1976.

This is by no means to suggest that possible applications of instant photography are limited to these patient populations, but rather, to point out

Portions of this chapter have been excerpted from the following articles:

The Polaroid Technique: Spontaneous Dialogues from the Unconscious. Published in *The International Journal of Art Psychotherapy*, Vol. 3, pp. 197-214, Pergamon Press, 1976 and also in *The Dynamics of Creativity*, (The annual proceedings of the American Art Therapy Association Conference, 1977), Barbara Mandel, Roberta Hastings Shoemaker, ATR, and Ronald Hayes, ATR, Editors. Robert Wolf, M.P.S., ATR, Author.

The Use of Instant Photography in the Establishment of a Therapeutic Alliance. Published in *Creativity and the Art Therapist's Identity*. (The Annual Proceedings of the American Art Therapy Association Conference, 1976), Roberta Hastings Shoemaker, ATR and Susan Gonick-Barris, ATR, Editors. Robert Wolf, M.P.S., ATR, Author.

Instant Phototherapy: Some Theoretical and Clinical Considerations for its Use in Psychotherapy and Special Education, By Robert Wolf, M.P.S., ATR. In *Phototherapy*, 1981, 3(1), pp. 3-6.

that the use of this technique is still in its infancy. However, since most of my experience has been gleaned from work with these populations, the content of this chapter will focus upon my theoretical understanding of the impact of instant photography upon the development of object relationships and ego skills, which are a central component of the therapeutic treatment of autism, learning disabilities and acting out behavior disorders.

I will also discuss the interrelationship between visualization and verbalization of affects, as promoted by our instant photo technique, and the effect of this process on the tendency to act out as often found in antisocial personalities.

WHY INSTANT PHOTOGRAPHS?

The instant photo is a spontaneous document. It captures the present in a "stop-action" form and offers to the viewer an opportunity to observe, examine and respond to what has just occurred. This quality of immediate feedback tends to hold the attention of the viewer, especially if he himself has taken or been the subject of the photograph. It offers him a nonthreatening way to take a close look at aspects of himself that previously may have been lost in the confusion of his impulsiveness. The photos can serve to initiate important discussions that may ultimately elicit significant information about the viewer. In therapeutic sessions this often leads to new energy and interest and can result in important insights in the patient.

The initial experience of having his own photo taken may also help a resistant patient overcome anxiety. It immediately engages him on a level at which he can feel personally involved in the therapy process. This investment holds the patient's interest and stimulates further involvement as the therapeutic relationship continues to evolve.

Even impulsive patients who require a great deal of structure and seek immediate gratification are able to utilize this technique because of the spontaneous nature of the instant print: they are figuratively held captive by the excitement of seeing their own image reflected in the photograph.

THE BASIC TECHNIQUE

The instant camera may be used in psychotherapy in a wide variety of ways. It may be used as part of a single diagnostic evaluation or as an integral part of long-term, ongoing psychotherapy (Wolf, 1978). Regardless of the manner of its use, however, I have found the following general procedure to be helpful. The procedure, of course, may be modified to suit a specific situation.

The therapist introduces an instant camera and film into the therapy session and demonstrates its use. Then he may suggest that he and the patient photograph each other. This can be expanded upon in several ways. The therapist may suggest that each person pretend to do something, make a silly face or gesture, or he may simply ask how the patient feels today and suggest that he give this feeling bodily or facial expression in the photo.

In a group, the therapist may suggest that photos be taken of group members. The selection process may be by group decision, or, depending upon the group's need for structure, may be left to the therapist alone.

After the photos are taken, the group or patient is instructed, with the therapist's help, to cut out the figures from their backgrounds. Next, photos selected by the patient are placed on a neutral paper in a configuration of his own design, and glued into place. The backgrounds as well as the figures may be used. The determination of how many figures or background photos will be used, or of their configuration on the paper, may be left to the patient or structured by the therapist.

The patient and therapist together look at the picture and begin to associate playfully to the images. The patient is encouraged to playfully draw in elements which elaborate his associations and begin to locate the photo-images in time and space. The negative space, created in the background pieces when the figures have been removed, may be drawn in by the therapist or the patient. New elements may be added by simple line drawings, paint, magic markers, cray-pas, etc. New images may also be added by taking new photos and creating a collage. The original images serve as a starting point and are often expanded in very creative ways by the patient.

For some patients this in itself may lead to significant new material for discussion with the therapist. Some less verbal youngsters may not be able to move to the next step described below. It is important for the therapist to be sensitive to the abilities and needs of each patient in determining how far to pursue this process.

If, however, the patient is able to work on a verbal level, it may be helpful for the therapist to ask him to look carefully at each element in the finished picture and envision himself as each figure. The patient is then asked to say whatever he feels the figure is saying, thinking or doing. These verbalizations may then be written verbatim, in cartoon caption format, by either the therapist or the patient.

If there is more than one figure in the picture, the therapist may elicit an ongoing dialogue from the patient by asking him to become each person and respond to the previous verbalization. This may go on until the patient is satisfied with the dialogue. The therapist may just help to document the patient's responses or may actively engage in the dialogue by taking on the role of one or more of the characters. This approach resembles the technique of psychodrama except that we now have created a lasting product of the imaginative experience to which the patient may later refer.

GRAPHIC ELABORATION: A PSYCHOANALYTIC PERSPECTIVE

We use the instant photo as a screen upon which the patients may project images and explore their underlying significance. This process is similar to the "free association" employed in traditional psychoanalysis. In the free association process, a patient is asked to assume a relaxed state and verbalize whatever thoughts, feelings or images enter his mind. These are then further explored by examining their latent content, that is to say, the underlying thoughts or feelings which link each of these elements together. Often it is not until the patient has carefully explored these underlying thoughts that the significance of the original images becomes clear.

In a similar way we ask our patients to "play" with their photos and draw whatever they wish to add or graphically elaborate upon to their original image. The therapist may then be able to help the patient explore the underlying content of these images and trace them back to emotionally significant issues. By creating a playful tone in the session the therapist is often able to help the patient overcome his resistance to this process.

Many elements of primary process thought may occur during this elaboration process. At first, time and space distortions and the recognition that many of his thoughts are connected by proximity or opposition to each other may be quite frightening to the patient. He doesn't know why he is drawing what he is! Here the therapist's ability to help him relax and play with the seemingly illogical material as it emerges is often crucial for the successful application of this technique.

Once a relaxing atmosphere is created, the therapist's instruction to cut the figures from their backgrounds may stimulate the patient's fantasy life. As the figure is freed from its links in time and space which had been provided by the background field of the photo, the patient can more easily focus on important nonverbal aspects of each figure. The body language, gestures and facial expressions which had been camouflaged by other, stronger reality elements of the photo, begin to emerge more vividly. This helps the patient to become more aware of and sensitized to the nonverbal elements of his images.

According to psychoanalytic theory, when certain emotions are not consciously experienced, they are not communicated through mechanisms that are consciously controlled. Because all emotions or affects do seek expression, nonverbal forms of communication such as gestures and physical stance, along with other more indirect forms of communication such as slips of the tongue, omissions and additions, often contain significant emotionally laden unconscious messages. So as the patient sharpens his ability to focus on these nonverbal elements and is encouraged to graphically elaborate on his images, he demonstrates how well this technique lends itself to the discovery of unconscious material.

Variations

The possibility for variations of this technique are often limited only by the therapist's reluctance to relinquish control over the structure of the session. We have found that some of the most creative applications of this technique were discovered by patients who were given the freedom to explore the range of possibilities without restriction.

This photo medium lends itself particularly well to the creation of finger puppets. The therapist may photograph the patient's face and hands and have them cut out and fastened to small rings of paper that can slip around one's fingers. You then have a spontaneous finger puppet that can be further embellished with found materials or just left as is. Children love to role play characters that they create in this manner. The therapist may easily make a puppet of himself as well and role play along with the patient. Reversing roles is quickly accomplished by exchanging puppets. As one may imagine, the projective potential of this kind of project is limitless.

Another interesting project with tremendous projective potential is the three dimensional stage. Figures are cut out and fastened in a free standing fashion to a piece of paper which acts as the floor in a scene of the patient's own design. He can add characters by photographing other people or posing for photos in various gestures. The patient can draw and add color directly to the photo to create the different characters. Imagine the potential for uncovering unconscious attitudes toward various family members if you ask a youngster to role play each family member and create representational characters out of their photographs! Additional material will of course come from the patient's placement of each figure.

There are various devices commercially available which can enhance these instant photo scenes. One is a clear plastic cup with space to insert artwork which can then be viewed through the transparent outer surface. Another is a badge-making kit that laminates artwork onto a metal button that can be worn on one's clothing. These materials are available through mailorder catalogs and motivate the patient to carry off, into his world, projects which represent his work and relationship with his therapist. This is particularly important when working with youngsters who tend to use the therapist as a transitional object and need to feel connected to him during the long hours which separate each session.

OTHER THEORETICAL ASPECTS

Ego Building Qualities

It is generally agreed that the ego develops from the infant's experience of his body. Ego psychologists have made much use of the concept that the ego is at first a body ego. This certainly makes good sense from a developmental perspective, for the young infant is immersed in a world of physical experiences. Sight, touch and sound are the first perceptions with which the growing infant begins to make sense out of the initially confusing bombardment of stimuli.

It is, therefore, understandable that an experience that focuses upon one's visual perception of oneself would help to strengthen ego weaknesses that have led to distortions in body image or self-concept. By providing a variety of visual feedback, the photo medium offers the patient an opportunity to organize his perceptions and ultimately learn who he is. It may be quite therapeutic for the patient to simply have a chance to observe how he looks from different perspectives.

In addition to these primary ego skills I have found this technique promotes the development of other ego skills as well. Organizational skills are stimulated as the patient learns to follow the simple tasks that are required by this procedure. He must learn to follow instructions, delay immediate gratification for the benefit of greater future satisfaction, and learn sequencing skills in order to operate the camera effectively. The patient also develops his integrative skills as he attempts to create an environment for his figures. By drawing in the fantasy background and adding other imaginative elements which locate the initial image in time and space, the patient begins to familiarize himself with certain of his unconscious and preconscious fantasies. Then in the process of talking about these images and ultimately their related feelings and conflicts, further integration of inner and outer aspects of the patient's personality is achieved. It is this "owning" of previously repressed or dissociated parts of the ego which fosters a strengthening process. Libidinal energy which was previously used in the service of repression is now freed for more productive purposes. It is important to note that for certain patients, particularly young children, this "owning" of fantasies may occur on a playful or symbolic level without the need for the patients to gain conscious insight into the historical root of the conflict. A resolution of the conflict may occur in this manner as the child gains a symbolic sense of mastery over his psychic dilemma and frees energy previously bound up in the struggle. The patient's abstracting skills are stimulated as he draws images which on some level relate to his inner life. The process of transformation from inner fantasy into an externalized two dimensional drawing promotes the patient's ability to perform abstract tasks. Further verbalizations continue to strengthen this bridge between abstract images and concrete thoughts, lending breadth and depth to the patient's sense of self.

Impact On Object Relationships

A second major area where I have found instant phototherapy to have significant impact is in the development of the patient's object relationships. By using this technique as an integral part of ongoing psychotherapy I have seen marked improvement in the patient's level of object relatedness. This is particularly important for patients who have had problems in their separation/individuation phase of development (Mahler, 1963).

The patient is thus able, in a playful manner, to work through his difficulty in differentiating between self and object — a major developmental task. Seeing himself and the therapist in various positions, at times by themselves, at other times together, he is slowly able to internalize the concept of feeling himself to be a separate, functioning person/object. Furthermore, by cutting out these figures and reintroducing them into self-created environments, the patient is allowed to develop a sense of mastery over this differentiation process.

Another important process which is promoted by using instant photos is the patient's ability to internalize his object representations. In other words, the patient may begin to take, inside of himself, a psychic representation of his therapist, which may then enable him to function more autonomously. By feeling as though he has the therapist (clearly representing the mother, transferentially) with him, he is more able to feel comfortable moving out into the world. This process may be compared to the concept of identification as a way to overcome a sense of object loss. Many youngsters who have been unable to successfully internalize representations of their own mothers in this fashion may discover a second chance to correct this handicap through this process. The therapist may offer to provide such a youngster with a creative journal which he may keep with him at home and bring to sessions with him. In this journal the youngster may glue photographs of himself and of the therapist. This journal may well become an important link between the therapist and patient, enabling the patient to slowly improve his ability to achieve object constancy and feel as though he is still in the presence of the therapist even during the days between actual sessions.

I have often found that the ability of children with learning disabilities to maintain a level of object constancy has been impaired by early environmental failures. Whether these failures are caused by defective responses by early objects or are a result of genetic predispositions or a combination of both is a debatable issue and one that extends beyond the scope of this paper. It is sufficient to say that whatever the cause, the fact remains that without this important developmental milestone having been reached, the youngster suffers in both his interpersonal relationships and, as I shall later discuss in greater detail, in his ability to cathect knowledge, or in other words, to learn! By offering photos of the therapist in this format we are providing a reparative process in which the journal may be used by the patient as a transitional object (Winnicott, 1975). The journal becomes highly cathectic and offsets the anxiety created by the transferential reconstruction of the original traumatic separation from the early object. Other theoreticians have described similar ways in which children ward off separation anxiety. Anna Freud described how young toddlers often go into a trancelike state which she calls "imaging" when separated from their mothers. In this "imaging" process she speculates that the infant conjures up an image of the lost mother and is then relieved of all anxiety.

On another level, patients with separation/individuation conflicts may be able to successfully resolve these conflicts by symbolically exploring, in a playful manner, their wish for fusion with the object and the concomitant fear of being engulfed by the object. Patients seem more able to explore these frightening parts of themselves through the use of their visual images. The atmosphere of playfulness offers a safe place within which visual images may be freely elicited and explored.

TREATMENT IMPLICATIONS

Defenses and Resistance to the Therapeutic Process

Visual images may often circumvent secondary process verbal defenses and lead us to highly cathected, libidinally charged unconscious conflictual material (Robbins, 1980). Through the ongoing use of instant phototherapy the therapist can get a clear pattern of the patient's defense mechanisms by listening to the secondary revisions which are used by the patient to move away from this conflictual material as it is inevitably stirred up. It is important to note that verbalizations may at times lead towards unconscious conflicts and at other times may lead away from them. The therapist must use his sensitivity and empathic skill to know whether a statement is authentic or defensive and encourage the patient to move in a direction which leads to a sense of self-awareness and integration. At times the therapist may enter the patient's world of images to make meaningful contact; he may enter the visual metaphor without attempting to analyze it. This may leave the patient with the sense of being deeply understood and appreciated, and foster a sense of therapeutic alliance.

Transference Assessment

Instant photos may be used to uncover patient's transference reactions to the therapist. The therapist needs only to suggest to the patient that he take a photo of the therapist and, as described above, draw in the background. This elicits a great deal of fantasy material related to the therapist. Whenever possible, care should be taken to encourage the patient to set up the pose of the therapist by demonstrating the gesture or facial expression which the therapist should assume for the photo. This tends to create an image of the therapist upon which the patient may easily project all kinds of fantasies. It is often helpful to do a transference assessment periodically to monitor the subtle changes in the patient's attitude toward the therapist.

INSTANT PHOTOTHERAPY WITH LEARNING DISABLED CHILDREN

Effects of Object Relationships on Cognitive Growth

In one of his early letters, Freud described his concept of memory as being integrally related to that which had previously been internalized by the infant as libidinally cathected conflicts and fantasies. His thesis was that, from all that one is exposed to, one selects and remembers that which is found to be of "interest." He saw this "interest" as a derivative of the libido that had been originally attached to this early infantile repressed material. He further speculated that what was of interest today, that is, what one has chosen to remember and focus attention upon, could be examined in the psychoanalytic process through the technique of free association and found to be a derivative of some long lost and repressed infantile conflict.

The implication here is important for anyone who attempts to address themselves to the special needs of learning disabled children. Freud is, in a sense, saying that one's basic quest for knowledge, or the libidinally cathected drive to learn and explore that which is unknown, is intimately tied to the rediscovery of that which has been at an earlier time "known" and then later lost within oneself (Freud, 1966).

Later object relations theoreticians have taken Freud's concept and developed it further by pointing out that it is specifically the early object relationships, that is the infant's first relationships with parenting figures usually experienced within the first few months of life, which provide a foundation for one's later manifest drive to pursue knowledge (Modell, 1977). This thesis rests upon a careful study of the interrelationship between one's ability to achieve object constancy, that is, to perceive an object and hold in one's mind a mental representation of the object, and one's later ability to cathect knowledge in the world. It is believed that the latter ability is dependent upon the former and is accomplished through a process whereby the early object cathexis is transformed into a drive to cathect knowledge, that is to say, redirected from the inner to the outer world and displaced from an object onto an idea, concept or thought.

It is believed that it is not only the child's ability to internalize this early object that influences his later learning process, but it is the quality of the early relationship with that object which will profoundly influence the child's attitudes toward learning. Winnicott (Deri, 1978) has described in detail the effect that the infant's relationship with his mother can have upon his later attitude toward exploration of the world. He believed that the young child internalizes his mother's attitude toward his exploration of the world. If the mother looked upon her child's assertive and independent strivings as exciting and good, and responded with enthusiasm and encouragement, then this attitude would be internalized by the infant, taken in as a prototype or model of how one's attempts at exploration and pursuing creative achievements will be met. He further proposed that this internalized attitude is later projected out onto the world and is felt by the child as he grows older, as a generalized anticipation of how his independent strivings and creative efforts in life will be met by the world. This of course includes one's quest for knowledge, and anticipation of how one's effort to learn and grow will be met.

Implications for Treatment of Learning Disabilities

I have been speaking of one's "attitude" toward learning as a drive derivative of early object relationships. Let us now reflect upon how one's drive to learn can influence a child's performance in school. The desire to gain knowledge and the pleasure one obtains from learning most certainly will affect a child's interest in classes, attention span and general motivation in school. It should be considered as a separate yet highly influential aspect of any learning difficulty. With many learning disabled youngsters there may well be a specific cognitive deficit. Unfortunately, when this child is evaluated for special educational needs, the cognitive problem is often targeted for remediation without this attitudinal factor being taken into account. These two factors are integrally interwoven and must be treated separately and concurrently. Even with youngsters who are seen primarily as cognitively impaired, there is almost always an underlying emotional reaction to the disability which will ultimately be reflected in a poor self-image.

As I have described earlier, instant phototherapy can help facilitate the development of certain basic ego functions. These functions can often influence the child's acquisition of cognitive skills. Additionally, the improvement in object relationships that the instant phototherapy promotes would stimulate the youngster's desire to utilize his newfound skills. Utilization of instant phototherapy along with other remedial treatment programs which address specific impairments has proven to be a most effective total treatment plan for learning disabled youngsters. It is not the acquisition of skill alone that is so crucial for these youngsters; it is their interest and excitement in learning which, in the end, will help motivate them to overcome handicaps and move on in their lives. To have a skill alone is not enough — you must also have the desire to use it.

Illustrative Case

Joe is a nine-year-old, learning disabled youngster seen in private art therapy treatment. He is currently enrolled in a special education school for emotionally handicapped, learning disabled youngsters. His younger brother is mildly mentally retarded, and his parents tend to deny their younger son's handicap and displace their anger and disappointment onto Joe. While there are soft signs of neurological deficits in Joe there is also a preponderance of emotional problems as characterized by immaturity, inability to relate to peers, impulsivity and lack of socialization skills. His major defenses of avoidance, denial, projection and projective identification imply a rather primitive level of emotional conflict. An elaborate treatment plan was formulated whereby Joe received intensive ongoing expressive art therapy while his family received occasional counseling on ways to help improve Joe's autonomous functioning and also to help them accept their younger son's handicap more easily.

Instant photography was introduced early in Joe's treatment and quickly became his central therapeutic modality. Joe responded well to the process. The therapist had to set clear firm limits around the number of photos that could be taken during each session. This helped Joe explore the potential of the modality while also helping to limit his impulsiveness. Without these limits Joe would have easily used up great quantities of film without much therapeutic progress.

One day the therapist took a photo of Joe as he posed with an angry expression on his face. Joe took the photo from the camera, waited for it to develop and created an interesting scene in which he is upset and afraid that a man named Stan "will get mad" if he, Joe, doesn't come up with an idea for a play. This example offers us an opportunity to observe how an instant photo may be utilized in ongoing therapy. First let us look at certain ego skills that are utilized in the process of creating this photo/drawing. Joe used his organizational skill to develop the photo, glue it to a paper and add a drawing which located the image in time and space. His capacity to integrate was expanded by the therapist's expectation for him to verbalize what the person is thinking, feeling or saying. As this theme is further explored, Joe begins to see, on a playful level, that he is feeling pressured to do something and complies out of fear that someone will be angry if he doesn't do what is expected. This visual image has enabled Joe to express heretofore hidden negative transference feelings. His father's disappointment in Joe's school functioning is openly expressed at home and is reexperienced in the treatment setting, through the transference, as his fear of making the therapist/father angry, by not being able to meet his expectations. To return to other ego skills, Joes ability to achieve abstract thought is stimulated by the task of visually representing his preconscious fantasies through drawings.

Other instant photos revealed some difficulty in differentiating between "self" and "object." One day Joe took a photo of the therapist and used it to draw a scene in which the therapist received an award for winning a pie-eating contest. He experiences the therapist as himself, struggling with the very same developmental conflicts as Joe himself struggles with. His oral wish to encorporate can be seen through the distortion of his defenses of denial and projec-

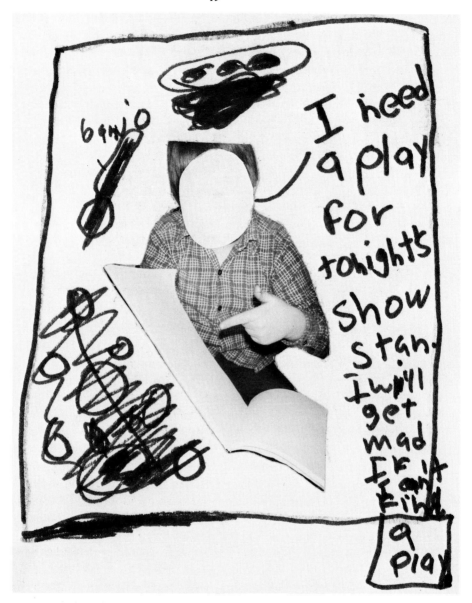

Figure 9-1.

tion. The conflict over the expression of this wish — if I devour the object which I need I will no longer have that object — is playfully expressed through the "accidental" cutting-off of the top of the therapist's head. This symbolic expresssion of a frightening conflict enabled Joe to slowly approach the previously threatening wish/fear and slowly begin to work it through. The playfulness of the creative art experience gave him a sense of safety as he explored the depths of these primitive feelings.

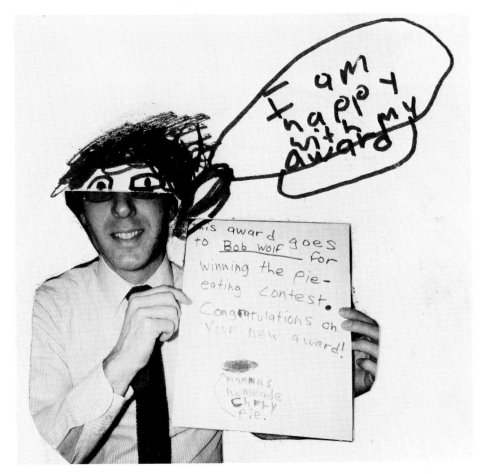

Figure 9-2.

Important underlying feelings are easily brought forward into the treatment setting through instant photos. During another session the therapist took a photo of Joe which he quickly took from the therapist and began to draw on. He decided not to cut out the background and instead glued the entire photo to a piece of drawing paper and spontaneously began to tell the therapist a story about "Crazy Arnie or The Boy Who Wanted to Die." The central theme was about a boy who gets sick and is saved by a doctor who brings magic pills for Arnie. The positive transference implications are quite clear here — he sees the therapist as a source of magical power and strength derived from oral supplies, but the underlying fear of being crazy and concurrent death wish was only briefly alluded to and had to be further explored, in greater detail by the therapist. Joe had used the instant photo as a messenger — he had sent out a call for help through it. In this way, the therapist was able to explore, with Joe, many of his most frightening feelings. As this process continued Joe began to

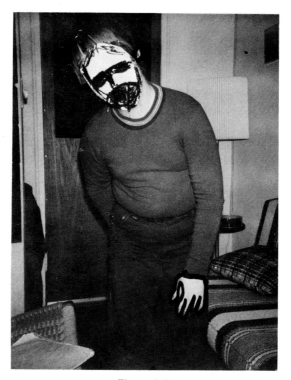

Figure 9-3.

show marked improvement in both his schoolwork and functioning with peers. He no longer assumed the role of the scapegoat with classmates. He was able to maintain friendships and began to demonstrate improvements in socialization skills. His academic work improved to the point where he was reevaluated by the local school board's evaluation unit and found to be ready for a less restrictive classroom setting.

INSTANT PHOTOTHERAPY WITH ACTING-OUT, ANTISOCIAL CHILDREN

Developmental Aspects of Acting-out Behavior

Recent studies into the root of acting-out and antisocial behavior have led to the identification of some factors that contribute to its manifestation (Rexford, 1978).

1. Early traumatic, and often repeated object loss.
2. Early parental attitudes in which the mother is experienced as ambivalent, unempathic and unpredictable as she inconsistently dealt with her child's anxieties and conflicts at each maturational phase;

especially during the first two years of life.

3. Continual parental encouragement of instinctual expression.
4. Overstimulation by the parents.
5. Disturbance in the maturational sequences of motor system and speech development.
6. A predisposition to action as a major mode of communication and reinforcement by the environment of this behavior.

Implications for Treatment of Acting-Out and Antisocial Disorders

As a result of these constitutional and environmental factors these children develop in a pathological way. They are often left with a deeply rooted belief that it is not worth pursuing relationships with anyone because people will inevitably disappear. Their identification with their mother's aggression and devaluation often leads to a disregard for and devaluation of themselves. The unpredictability of their early environment along with their own heightened tendency toward nonverbal, visual communications leads to a hyperalertness to looking at or being looked at. Because of their early traumatic object losses they usually experience deficiencies in achieving object constancy. This is seen as being intimately tied to their inability to delay discharge of tension and low tolerance of anxiety. With this understanding of the underlying dynamics behind these manifest behavioral problems, let us now look at how instant phototherapy may be utilized to help these youngsters overcome their handicap.

These youngsters are literally stuck at an early developmental level of object relations. They are fixated at the level of primary narcissism where their libidinal energy is turned inward upon themselves. Their traumatic experiences with frustrating and frightening objects has left them fearful of attempting to invest libidinal energy in anyone other than themselves. Yet they are hypersensitive to nonverbal, visual stimuli. Here is where we can make contact.

With instant photographs we can begin to take pictures of these children and "stop" their action. This offers them an opportunity to view their own actions with new scrutiny. Being so sensitive to nonverbal cues, because they never knew how their parent would react from minute to minute, they can study their own gestures and expressions in the photos. Slowly, the therapist can encourage the child to verbalize what he sees. This process begins to build up the child's verbalization skills and helps to connect him to his feelings. It helps to provide an alternate method of expression of feelings. As the child learns that the therapist responds to verbal expression of feelings, the previous drive toward motoric expression may be modified. As the child begins to photograph the therapist and identify with him as a more benign, supportive and consistently available object, he is able to modify the destructive effects of his earlier identifications with his sadistic parent. As this transformation process proceeds, he is able to begin to redirect his narcissistic libido onto a new object — the therapist. This achievement helps to bind destructive impulsive urges and reduce autoerotic activity, freeing energy with which he may now more easily explore the world around him.

This transformation process is a slow one. The therapist must be prepared to bear the brunt of these children's ambivalent feelings as they are manifest in the transference. The early traumas will inevitably be reexperienced, by the patient, as treatment progresses. Firm boundaries must be set along with a feeling tone of tolerance and empathic understanding. The therapist must view these "affect-storms" as a positive prognostic sign. The patient should be able to displace some of these destructive affects into his photo/artwork and take distance from these feelings when necessary. The therapist must use his sensitivity to know when to push the patient toward feeling these affects and when it is more helpful to allow this displacement to occur. As a result of this process, the child is led through a reparative emotional experience where he gains renewed hopefulness: he learns that human relationships don't have to be disappointing; that not all people are totally unpredictable and pursuit of human contact may, in fact, lead to warm and gratifying experiences.

What I am proposing here is that the therapist must find a route of intervention into the world of an acting-out child. His suspiciousness and deeply rooted fear of genuine contact make the acting-out child quite difficult to reach, but his hyperalertness to visual and nonverbal communication, along with his covert drive for contact and hunger for more positive kinds of identifications, make him an ideal candidate for instant phototherapy. His narcissistic fixation also helps to anchor him in the treatment process when the therapist begins the treatment by taking photos of the patient.

THE USE OF INSTANT PHOTOTHERAPY
IN HELPING TO ESTABLISH A THERAPEUTIC ALLIANCE

Before any meaningful treatment can occur you must first gain the trust of and form a sense of alliance with your patient. This seemingly simple statement may be quite difficult to accomplish if you work with patient populations demonstrating psychopathic, antisocial or acting-out character disorders. The problem with these patients is that they often do not believe that they need help or that they, indeed, have any problems. Most often they are remanded for treatment, often by the court, and agree to engage in a treatment process only as a way to get what they ultimately want — to be back on the street, continuing their antisocial endeavors without getting caught. They are very often masters at manipulation and can easily fool a neophyte therapist into believing in their sincere effort to reform, when, in fact, they simply desire to use the therapist for their own purposes without any deep belief that they are in trouble and need professional help (MacKinnon and Michels, 1971). They are not able to tolerate anxiety or tension and tend to bolt from treatment at the first sign of these painful affects. This is, of course, another manifestation of their tendency toward action as a primary mode of discharge of affect. This poses a difficult treatment/management issue. For whenever the therapist begins to probe any affect-laden material, the patient will acknowledge this noble effort by attempting to run away!

What must first take place is the development of a sense, by the patient, that the therapist is a friend; someone who truly cares in a real way, and will be there in a consistent and empathic way to try to help connect the patient to his feelings and explore the manifestations of his acting-out in a nonjudgmental way, while at the same time, creating a sense of structure and accountability which the patient must respect and function within. In other words, the anticipation is that there will be acting-out within the treatment parameters, yet it will be expected that the patient and therapist will explore its meaning and try to unravel the mystery of its manifestation with the ultimate hope that this process can be expanded to include all forms of acting-out in the patient's life.

As described earlier, the level of narcissistic fixation in these patients, and their hyperalertness to visual, nonverbal cues make a nonverbal form of treatment desirable. Often, it is important to begin treatment with an initial period of getting to know each other. Taking instant photos of each other can provide an initial bridge, through which the therapist may begin to make contact. During this treatment phase, the therapist conveys the sense of structure (by being on time and expecting the patient to come consistently) and talks of the need for the patient's support in this process.

Illustrative Case

Lester is a thin, frail seventeen-year-old youth of Jamaican descent. Although his family was extremely poor and lived in a condemned tenement, he always managed to dress impeccably, in the most contemporary fashions. He was referred for treatment as a last resort before discharge because of his increasing involvement in antisocial activities. After a period of marginal adjustment to a special education junior high school, he had been involved in the theft of office equipment from the school. The burglary was accompanied by an unusual degree of vandalism. Furniture had been overturned, papers strewn about and ink spilled over everything. This violence did not fit with Lester's outwardly friendly and compliant manner.

He made two drawings on the day following the burglary. In the first, everything was separate; often incomplete. Size and proportion were irrelevant; one got the feeling that things didn't really relate to each other. In much the same way, Lester didn't relate to people in life. The second drawing displayed a conspicuous absence of people: the world is unreal, objects

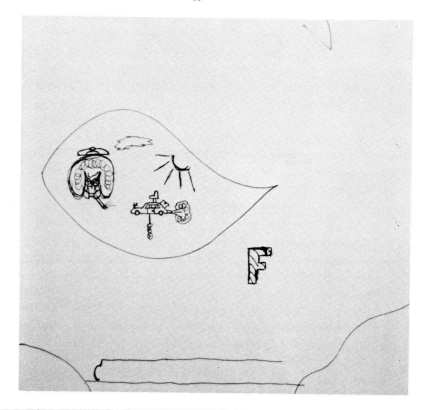

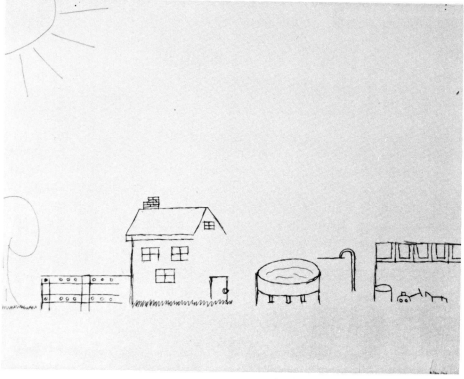

Figure 9-4 a and b.

floating, nothing is connected to the ground or to each other. One gets the feeling that if all the lines were to connect and the forms were brought into relationships with each other, it would be impossible to hide from the emptiness and pain of this world. This would be too devastating for Lester. At this point he needed these defenses to protect his fragile sense of self which lay beneath his cool facade.

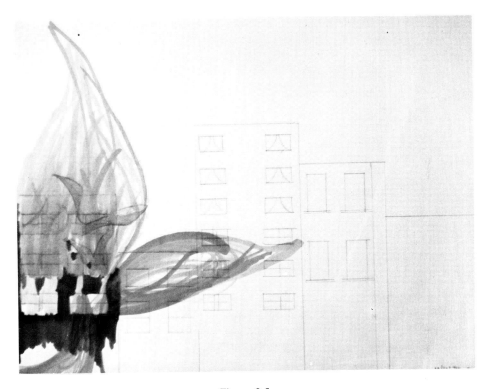

Figure 9-5.

Our initial contacts soon became too threatening for him. His next drawings of rigid tenements were made with rulers. During the second session he began to draw one house on fire and became so anxious that he had to leave the office. He was not ready for such a direct approach. His feelings had begun to break through his rigid, crumbling defenses and he sought the only other means of defense he knew — motoric discharge. He just left! We needed to find a slower approach which would permit him to strengthen his sense of self and encourage him to build a trusting relationship with his therapist. Only then would he perhaps be able to withstand the anxiety which mounted as he became more connected to his feelings.

It was at this point, where Lester was asking for help yet unable to utilize traditional verbal therapy, that I offered him an instant camera and suggested that we together make a scrapbook of his neighborhood; taking photos and pasting them into a book or onto posters.

Until this point it had been difficult to motivate Lester and stimulate his interest for any period of time but with the instant photo medium, his sense of mastery, immediate gratification and feeling of being in control of his environment worked together to engage him in this project for several weeks. The collage posters were designed by Lester and constructed entirely from instant photos which we had taken while walking together through his neighborhood. During this period we spent much time out of the special education school setting and roamed about together, exploring his world, talking about almost anything, and just getting to know each other. By using the camera he was able to reenter his home/environment and focus on its elements; examining them with new curiosity and objectivity. He would notice new things and see old things in new ways. This process slowed down his motoric activity and further stimulated his visual perceptual ability.

At first he photographed only inanimate objects. He seemed to get pleasure out of taking 'inventory' of his world. He was confirming his reality; separating fact from fantasy. After a while he began to take interest in photographing people. We entered a phase where all he wanted to do was photograph me and have me photograph him. We did this for some time — taking photos of each other in various positions and in many different places. He was allowing himself to begin to experience people in his world. Up until this point it was too frightening for him to really relate to anyone, but slowly, as trust began to build in our relationship, he was able to overcome this fear and his underlying hunger for human contact began to appear. We spent the last few minutes of each session reviewing the daily photos and when we had enough to mount he would carefully paste them onto his posters or into his scrapbook. Many of these projects were taken home or brought to classes for teachers or friends to view as a constant reminder of his growing ability to maintain contact in a highly gratifying relationship.

This nonthreatening, ego strengthening activity gave Lester the opportunity to develop his aesthetic ability as well. He took great pride in his work. A new playfulness began to emerge as he proposed silly poses for our photos. This seemed to tap into a wealth of creativity which had previously been blocked behind his cool facade. He began to take greater interest in his academic work. As he began to realize his creative resources, he was able to apply this to his academic studies, particularly science, social studies and creative writing. Lester began to show signs of identification with his therapist. Identification, being an unconscious process, is strongly affected by nonverbal experience. Having so many photos of himself and his therapist helped him to build a connection to his therapist which offered an important new foundation for his growing yet tenuous personality. This new model was seen as warm, caring and consistent, yet at times also confrontive and firm. As Lester slowly internalized

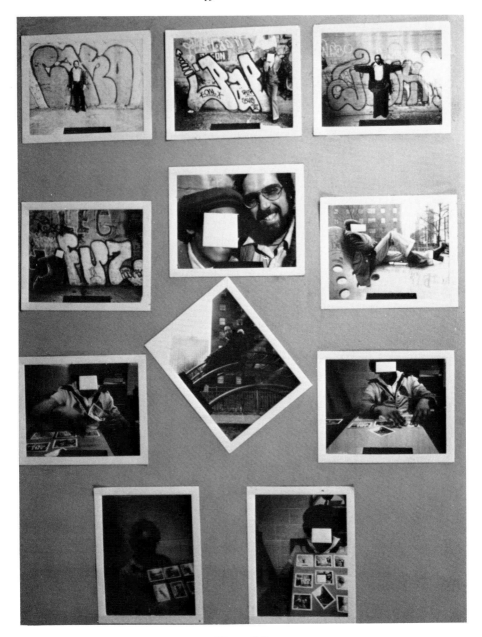

Figure 9-6.

this new model he was able to free himself from the destructive effects of other previous more pathological or toxic introjects. Quite spontaneously he one day proposed that we begin a new series of projects. He wanted to return to work in the office and create a series of drawings and poems. He had been able to develop sufficient trust in me to neutralize the anxiety that had previously in-

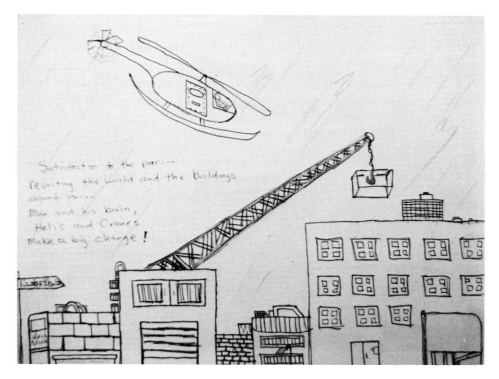

Figure 9-7.

terfered with our working together in such close proximity.

He was able to draw freely and write about whatever thoughts or images he experienced. These drawings were in marked contrast to his earlier rigid, constricted work.

One of his last drawings was made at the end of the school year. It was a city scene. In striking contrast to the unreal first drawings of almost one year ago, this scene was more solid, grounded and connected. Behaviorally, his acting out had stopped and he was functioning well in school. He was well liked by his classmates and was able to express himself more freely both verbally and artistically, through words, poems and drawings.

REFERENCES

Deri, S.: Transitional Phenomenon: Vicissitudes of Symbolization and Creativity. *Between fantasy and reality.* New York: Aronson, 1978.

Freud, S.: Letter #52. *Standard Edition.* London: Hogarth, *1*:233, 1966.

Gee, E. N.: Play, Art And Photography In A Therapeutic Nursery School. *Creative Art Therapy.* New York: Brunner-Mazel, 1976.

MacKinnon, R.A. and Michels, R.: *The psychiatric interview in clinical practice.* Philadelphia: Saunders, 1971.

Mahler, M.: Thoughts About Development And Individuation. *The Psychoanalytic Study Of The*

*Child, XVIII:*307, 1963.

Modell, A.: *Object love and reality.* New York: International Universities Press, 1977.

Rexford, E.: *A developmental approach to problems of acting out.* New York: International Universities Press, 1978.

Robbins, A.: *Expressive therapy: A creative arts approach to depth oriented treatment.* New York: Human Sciences Press, 1980.

Winnicott, D.W.: Transitional Objects And Transitional Phenomenon. *Through paediatrics to psychoanalysis.* New York: Basic Books, 1975.

Wolf, R.: The Polaroid Technique: Spontaneous Dialogues From The Unconscious. *The International Journal Of Art Psychotherapy, 3:*197, 1976.

Wolf, R.: Creative Expressive Therapy: An Integrative Case Study. *The International Journal Of Art Psychotherapy, 5:*81, 1978.

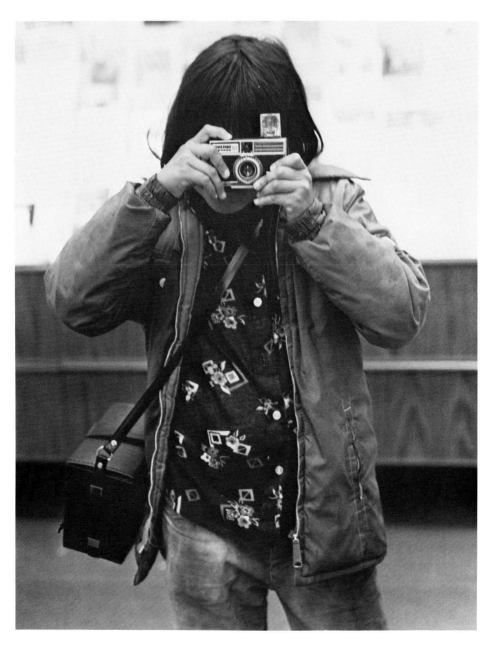

Chapter 10

Using Photographs in Therapy with People Who are "Different"

JUDY WEISER

INTRODUCTION

"HOW many people are in this picture?" asks the recent advertisement for the International Year of the Disabled. There are ten, two of whom are in wheelchairs. Apparently most viewers see only the eight on foot as "people." Being invisible, skipped over, talked around, patronized, and given little credit for individuality are common occurrences for disabled people, and their families often get caught up in it as well. Similar things happen to those from other cultures or races that are in minority status, or even to "invisible" members of a family or group who may be for whatever reason in disfavor--i.e. people who are "different."

Using a systems theory model of approach, one quickly realizes that a group or family with a disabled or "different" member really is a nonentity, rather, the term "disabled or different group/family" is more appropriate — because *all* persons in that system are affected by one member's entry into the category of handicapped/disabled, or by their standing out as somehow different than the majority. *All* persons will to some degree readjust, shift, change their expectations, thoughts, hopes, dreams, attitudes, feelings, and sometimes even their very methods of communication with an individual who does not fit the common mold.

For example, therapists often encounter such families as part of the rehabilitation process, in the midst of the immediate crisis, with family members as well as the identified problem/disabled client going through stages of dealing with the disability that are very similar to the stages of facing and grieving a death. Similarly, multicultural groups and communities deal with the continuum between treating everyone the same versus honoring and respecting differences (even though those differences may lead to lack of consensus or demands for specialized treatment). Such groups may find themselves stuck for solutions when the differences seem polarized or unexplainable to others.

Families or communities that have "adjusted," on the other hand, are rarely encountered by the helping professionals, unless for reasons apart from the disability or differentness. Assisting people to reach the "adjusted" stage, to learn to understand and accept and respect people, to separate the real differences-that-make-a-difference (societal and cultural as well as physical and emotional) from the sham excuses (without those differences being seen as threatening), to cope and yet go on to maintain a "healthy" relationship — these are some of the goals of therapists, and there are many standard methodologies of reaching these goals, usually dependent on purely verbal interactions.

One of the seemingly newer helpful techniques — though actual earliest documentation places it at roughly 1857 — is phototherapy, a catch-all phrase describing the use of the process of taking pictures and looking at pictures, as well as the product of the photo/print itself (and what one does with it), as effective tools to add to the repertoire of skills a competent therapist draws from as ways to reach clients and assist their desired growth and change. Phototherapy is *not* a bounded set of rules and steps which one must follow in some order "or else. . .," nor is it some gimmicky "new-therapy-of-the-year"; rather it is an open-ended collection of methods that allow therapists and clients access to previously blocked areas of feelings, thoughts, attitudes, memories, etc., that had been otherwise unavailable through ordinary verbal means of counseling. These adjuncts to therapy are especially useful with those for whom the usual verbal channels of interaction and expression are not available, either physically (such as hearing-impaired, cerebral palsied, autistic, mentally retarded, aphasic, stroke-damaged, etc.) or emotionally or culturally (different languages, traditions, etc.), though certainly in no way limited to just these specific types. They work equally well for the nondisabled or the cultural majority, as they do for people who might not even be in therapy who simply want to explore how much they can learn about themselves from photos and their reactions to them.

The following pages will review some of the implications of being different in our society and explore in one case study the uses and possibilities of implementing phototherapeutic techniques (and the results that ensued).

BEING "DIFFERENT"

One is usually born into one's race — and one's culture grows with the person, most traditions and patterns well established in early childhood. Even if surrounded by "outsiders," there is usually a small unit (family or group) where one can retire into from the outside world, where one can be "normal" and accepted, be "just like everyone else." While this is personally reassuring, it reinforces the existence (and validity) of those differences which set the person apart from the majority. Just as a family must learn to respect and appreciate individual members' differences and differentness without these being seen as threatening to the continuation of the family's identity as a special unit, so must a society tolerate and value its various cultures and races without fearing them as somehow harmful (and thus demanding assimilation). Such attempts to change other races or cultures into what they aren't (such as demands and expectations pushed upon Native Indians or immigrants) are not only confusing to those individuals, but deadly to their self-esteem and pride as they lose their sense of continuity and respect for their own culture and its roots. They find that who they are is not good enough; they are expected to change (and to desire to change) even when they cannot comprehend the demands being made — and those demands are often unspoken, subtle, not shared with them.

A person from a minority race or culture who successfully "passes" loses part of himself while he gains the new acceptance and its freedoms that which set him apart, made him different and made him all right to be different sifts away, and people in these "marginal" statuses (straddling the line with one foot in each culture, usually trying to expand to keep both), often lose touch with who they are, and frequently encounter feelings of *angst* and alienation, of being out of touch with who they "really" are.

Growing up in a family where one member has always been disabled is in many ways similar to living with a person of another race or culture. One learns naturally which differences make a difference, and which don't matter (and which only matter to outsiders). The differentness is usually so much a part of normal life that it ceases to be noticed until situational limitations refocus attention. But this natural process is not similarly available to those who are suddenly disabled (or those who relate to such a person).

Becoming a disabled person is a major life change. People are expecting to have to cope with the bodily alterations, but they rarely are fully prepared for the onslaught of all the complex psychological factors that descend upon their lives. The steps of coming to terms with the "new" person are very similar to going through the stages of grief as described by Kübler-Ross (1975) and others: When someone you love dies, you have a feeling of numbness, a yearning, and a protest. You have lost part of yourself; you feel disorganized; and you do much crying. You are restless and you may feel guilty. Perhaps you could have helped, but you do not know how. You are angry because the person died, and you are angry at the world. You feel so alone, and loneliness is one of the biggest problems of grief. It is your problem and you have to solve it alone. One could easily substitute "disability" for "death" in the above passage. Similarly, being alone in a foreign culture can be equally alienating and frustrating.

People long experienced in work with disabled persons and families find it often helps to distinguish between *impairment* (any departure from normal functioning), *disability* (significant inability to perform a function considered useful, in spite of corrective measures), and *handicap* (the additional social dimension, including values, attitudes of self and others, legal restrictions, and technological/physical considerations such as architectural barriers, prostheses, etc.) (Freeman, 1981). One may well be handicapped with one group and not another; handicapping circumstances may not even be physiological in nature, as those in racial or cultural minorities would be able to concur.

If one or more attributes reduces a person from a whole and usual person to a discounted one, this discrediting attribute is a "stigma" (Freeman, 1981), and these can be cultural or racial as well as physical. Those with a stigma depart from usual expectations and are often seen to be not quite human, and thus subject to discrimination, deliberate or unintended. There is sometimes a "spread of stigma" to include those around the disabled or "different" person, and it is important to assess and deal with this situation. The siblings may also be affected, and quite sensitive especially in adolescence. Feelings can range; including resentment, anger, jealousy, guilt, fear, shame, and/or embarrassment, and there is frequently an accompanying lack of factual knowledge (Freeman, 1981). Similar reactions can be noted in classrooms and groups when a "different" child is brought in. People's sequence of responses to disability or close encounters with persons of a different race or culture depends upon whether the change is a surprise or not, but may include denial, shock, guilt, despair, and intellectualization and rationalization. Long-term effects of such an intrusion are complex, but in general divorce and separation are not any more frequent; a bad marriage may be worsened, however; and acceptance does not automatically mean serenity. The impact of a handicapped child into a family system may or may not mean a crisis for that family depending on the nature of the event, the resources of the family, and how the family itself defines the event. Likewise the introduction of a racially or culturally different person into any group can vary in consequence. It is not universally perceived as terrible to become disabled or be "different," and the degree of the crisis, if there indeed is one, is not always in direct proportion to the severity of the handicap.

The parents of handicapped children may find few of the typical joys that compensate for the frustrations and inconveniences imposed by their child. Dreams and hopes regarding the child's future are often shattered. The child who was to represent the extension of the parents' egos serves instead as a deflation of their egos. He or she may serve as a threat to the parents' self-esteem and feelings of self-worth and dignity, and they may view themselves as failures in what they consider one of their most fundamental purposes in life (Chinn, Winn, and Walters, 1978). Thus the satisfactions and successes of the handicapped child are often overlooked and overshadowed by frustrations that parents experience. Often it is the support system (family, group, or agency) that has the worst crisis, and they also need to be helped to recognize that there are indeed positive and satisfying experiences to be appreciated in their situation. Parallel complexities are encountered in adoption of a minority or mixed-race child.

Social competence involves certain skills; if children who are different do not have opportunities to move out from a secure base to explore relationships, they are likely to be skill deficient (Freeman, 1981). As Turner-Hogan (1981) comments in her phototherapeutic work with orthopedically handicapped teens, the adolescents who are physically handicapped often experience special difficulties in accomplishing the emotional tasks of this developmental stage. Specifically, the development of a positive self-image as a peer and as a near-adult is often impaired by negative self concepts (stemming from physical disability or perception of inferiority).

The way one adapts to a stigma becomes part of the stigma itself. Social expectations strongly influence social interactions; usually these are taken for granted, but when highly visible people are present, the situation is changed (Freeman, 1981). Similar to immigrants in a new and perplexing country, the disabled (while also readjusting to new limits and expectations, as well as often to a new body image) may fear loss of their place in their family and what part they will now be able to contribute. They become very finely tuned to "differences-that-make-a-difference," and indeed this can overmagnify what used to be unimportant comments and reactions into significant issues. People *do* need to have honest feedback as to how they are seen by others; attempts to cushion the effects only serve to delay autonomy. Attention should be paid to grooming, appearance, and habits that could adversely affect relationships (Freeman, 1981). And, it may be added, this desensitization is necessary not only for the client and his or her family, but also for budding therapists, teachers, etc. It is often easier for the professionals than for the family, as they are not as deeply or personally involved. Their involvement is usually by choice — if the work is not palatable, it can be discontinued. The parent, on the other hand, faces the child every day and night; the child that is in some way handicapped is a reality for the rest of the parents' lives (Chinn, Winn, and Walters, 1978). There is little we professionals can say or do to comfort; we are used to seeking "cures" with clients and families — disabling circumstances such as these, on the other hand, are things we cannot fix; they won't go away, no matter how hard we try.

People in distress cannot see beyond themselves. Additionally, their self-images have become distorted. They are blinded to some degree by their pain. Their perceptual mechanisms are not functioning fully, and they are left with a fairly frozen point of view and occluded ability to make fuller, larger, and more complete meanings from what they do see (Krauss, 1981). Thus the therapists' goals should aim toward expanding, with the client's active participation, the options and alternatives available and working on exploring them. Therapists must help clients to recognize the dimensions of what they are going through, that there are fairly universal stages and conditions that they will pass through (at their own speed), and that they will be going through similar emotions to those that other people have experienced and survived.

There is no single reaction to disability; families must recognize attitudes and feelings such as frustration, hurt, guilt, and despair, and be willing to honor them even if all members are not experiencing the same things at the same time. Each individual proceeds at his or her own pace through the various stages, sometimes linearly, sometimes several simultaneously, sometimes becoming stuck or blocked at one or many; each person's path being his or her own unique need to explore feelings through to acceptance in some form. Not everyone completes the process, nor do all go through all the stages. Most, once they are aware of and recognize a problem, go through some process of searching for a cause and a cure, dealing with their feelings along the way as they discover there is none, and finally in some manner accept the status quo.

Most parents of handicapped children go through feelings of defensive denial, projection of blame, hostility, fear, anxiety, confusion over the unknown, guilt, mourning, sadness, withdrawal, rejection. Reactions toward unexpected intrusion of minority races and cultures are frequently similar. People react to such things in a number of ways, including strong underexpectations of achievement where they devalue abilities (and encourage self-fulfilling prophesies), setting unrealistic goals (high) where failure can justify negative feelings and encourage continuing dependency, escape (physical, such as desertion, abandonment, or avoidance; or emotional), or a form of reaction formation where they publicly show affection and acceptance but do not really feel it (Freeman, 1981).

Learning how to cope with cultural or physical differences or change, to grow beyond their limitations, is the basis for therapy with such persons and their families. Clients need to be encouraged to the point that they see that being different is all right as long as they can successfully understand and handle the consequences. But at this point problems in the therapeutic process itself frequently arise.

THERAPY WITH THOSE WHO ARE "DIFFERENT"

Most models of training helping professionals stress the many varied procedures of engaging clients in "meaningful dialogue." Ease of communication and facility with the language used by the therapist are usually unchallenged assumptions; for example, many texts congratulate themselves for suggesting interpreters be used to exchange one language for another when difficulties arise — as if it is only the sounds of the words that are causing the confusions (rather than the entire cultural system and thinking structures those words represent). Some training is occasionally provided under the categories of international or cross-cultural studies, but it is rarely stressed that these concepts apply equally well to the "foreigners" among us, people we encounter in our daily lives who somehow "don't fit," clients we somehow cannot get through to with our ordinary linear verbal means of counseling. We think we make sense; they agree. We make suggestions that seem logical and call the client "resistant" when they are not carried out as we expected. We get a gut-level feeling sometimes that although verbally they seem to comprehend, they are not really with us. Their bodies are compliant, but their minds seem to be confused in ways that they do not even know how to express. Therapists seek progress toward the mutually agreed-upon goals; communication at all stages of this process is essential. When clients either cannot or will not relate to us through our ordinary verbal therapeutic process, we must have alternative tools that are based more on *their* own way of comprehending or communicating; phototherapy techniques provide such tools.

In its most basic form, communication is an agreement that perceptions and understandings can truly be shared, and it is nonverbal as well as verbal. It is the *agreement* itself, the consensus, the feeling that another person has grasped in the same way that we intended it, just what we meant them to grasp. Communication is *not* just words that mean exactly the same thing to every person regardless of context or the very act of perception. Misunderstandings can and frequently do occur when the same "reality" gives different messages to different people (especially if they do not realize this and proceed to act on what they perceive to be mutual agreement). As Bandler and Grinder (1979) and others are fond of saying, the map is *not* the territory itself; although it is very difficult to get families in crisis to comprehend this concept (because each person is certain that he or she knows how things really are at home), the realization of what it means and implies can be the watershed point of breakthrough for the therapy process. People think that what they perceive *truly* exists, and the criteria for judging such truth ("knowing") exists in them based in part on very early conditioning as to what they will and will not accept according to the values of their society (which is very much structured by the nature of that culture's linguistic categorization system and its expression).

It is all so deeply ingrained that the person usually cannot comprehend its subconscious and yet subjective nature, and therefore often finds any alteration of such concepts to be somewhat threatening (and therefore "wrong"). How people perceive their world appears to directly define it for them; their perceptions (and their biases) reflect their enculturation and affect the ways they will behave based on these assumptions. Thus when faced with relating to someone of radically differently values or perceptual modes, a person is often at a loss as to how to deal at all in this situation, and this usually results in perception of some threat which is quickly followed by fear and hostility. If people could only become more comfortable with the idea that theirs is not the *only* way to see things (but that it is *just* as valid as any other), and feel secure in this enlarged conceptual ideology, then interpersonal communication on small or large scale could be so much more easily facilitated. Using photographs, projectively and otherwise (as demonstrated elsewhere in this book), to serve as stimuli for people's responses serves as an excellent tool to see how differently we all see the "same" thing. Each person is "right" for himself or herself; there is no "wrong" way to experience a photograph. This can serve as a beginning step in communication.

Perception deals with differences that make a difference — in Gestalt terms, the figure that stands out from the ground; as we describe things, we bring into being ("existence") those things which are then later accepted as "real." For example, Eskimo people have dozens more terms for snow than we more southerly city-folk — separating out the subtle nuances that make a difference to them (which we would not even notice as differences) and could be a life-or-death matter; whereas for us, all those different categories do not exist at all. As another example, very young children do not comprehend a question asking what color their playmates are, but by the first few years of school, racial and cultural prejudices they have been taught are noticeable, and they begin to notice differences "which weren't there before." This has serious implications for therapy, where families or groups may be operating with individual members in different perceptual systems and not even know it, and then become frustrated when "natural" assumptions are not automatically shared. (Think, for example, of arguments between parents and children about appropriate dress for an occasion, or proper haircuts).

There really is no "right" or "wrong" existing all by itself in this world; only "different" — we, through our personal, societal, and cultural applications add the values that label, in both verbal and nonverbal form. Each of us imposes our own map; we are our own selective filters. The grave error is made when we think that what we perceive is some shared and universal reality existing itself apart from us, forgetting the effect of our perceptions, words, and symbols.

As Krauss (1981) has described the socialization process, living in any given culture teaches us a great deal about how we "should" experience the world. This "should" influences what we attend to and/or disregard in our environment; this is that society's process of training us as to what is deemed acceptable and what is unacceptable, what is real and what is not, and how the real may be experienced and understood. Additionally, as Krauss (1981) suggests, socialization thus involves the teaching of a specific orientation about "how to be" in the world as well as "that's the way it is." Each person who tries to help guide or teach (or "therapize") another person *must* recognize that their position is not intrinsically better or right; it is only a different one, one that happens to be in majority favor at that time. Deciding to change another person must take into account the opening up of options, not just the exchange of one closed system for another. And although it has been elsewhere mentioned in this book, it should be repeated that photographs of a group or culture are invaluable aids to understanding the "shoulds," the "acceptables," the "reals" for those people — their values and expectations are usually very clearly presented in what they choose to photograph and how they present themselves to the photographer.

And lastly in this section on theoretical implications in work with people who are "different," we must consider the implications from research into brain hemispheric lateralization. In short, researchers have found that the two halves of the brain, while extremely similar in appearance, are activated and involved in two different kinds of functioning. In is not an image of one side "on"/one side "off," but rather a continually shifting scale of differing proportions depending on what is on what is happening. The left brain is most involved when the person is engaged in analytic, sequential, categorical, rational, and usually verbally oriented thinking (we may have just described traditional therapy. . .). Left brain thinking is easily dichotomised into polarities with no middle ground: good/bad, on/off, right/wrong, yes/no. The right brain becomes more active when doing spatially oriented tasks, holistic, conceptual, integrative, intuitive, and metaphoric thinking, synthesizing gestalts, dreaming, imaging (and possibly idiogrammatic languaging), symbolizing, the more artistic endeavors, and usually the nonverbal and more emotional concepts of life and communication. People who are of a more right-brain dominant orientation would have trouble with simple dichotomies, seeing instead all the "gray areas" in between the more simplistic black or white polarities. For those readers familiar with computer terminology, the concept would be left brain = digital; right brain = analog. For those students of cultural anthropology, one could easily generalize Western Hemisphere cultures (such as the U.S.) more left-brain oriented, whereas the Eastern cultures (such as Japan) are more right-brain oriented; and their languages reflect this difference, as do the whole conceptual frameworks of their societies (for example, their orientations toward time concepts). It may seem perhaps a bit too simplistic, but one could possibly see it as a difference between thoughts and feelings, or verbal and nonverbal. A photograph itself could be seen as a right-hemisphere type of concept — a gestalt that is far more than just a list of "what's in the photo" (although inseparable from them), verb and noun all-at-once; never could a verbal explanation totally describe one of the feelings that accompany a photo, no more than one could do with a dream one had.

People who are most healthily "adjusted" seem to move easily between these two styles of orientation, whereas being blocked in one or the other can lead to difficulties (especially when trying to communicate with someone locked into the other). Therapists encounter such blocks frequently when working with people who are "different" (though they may not realize it consciously); often these are the very things about them that make them seem different! An example from my case experience is teenagers from either the deaf or Native Indian cultures, which are both primarily right-brain in orientation, with flexible rules and tolerances and attitudes towards things like time schedules and promptness, trying to fit into hearing people's or white society's more left-brain dominated system of rules, laws, "oughts," "shoulds," and "can'ts," especially with their strict values regarding time and being on time. Right-brain kids in a left-brain world; no wonder there is so much confusion between the cultures — people think they are all perceiving the same world the same way, and cannot figure out who or what to blame when differences arise. This obviously has implications for therapy, especially those methods that rely on primarily verbal and left-brain types of interaction, especially when they are used with clients who primarily are not! And this is exactly why phototherapeutic techniques can often work better, especially for those not fitting the stereotypical molds of the majority.

Too often we are too quick to judge clients as uncommunicative or unable to clearly communicate when it is ourselves who are handicapped by our lack of innovation to try something different, something out of the ordinary that just might work, precisely *because* of its differentness. In the pages that follow, readers will see application of phototherapeutic techniques to reach and help a client whose presenting diagnosis had been "unapproachable, uncommunicative, unfeeling, and probably retarded," various techniques overlaid, sometimes many at once, to implement the therapeutic consequences of the concepts discussed on the previous pages, for a client for whom the usual verbal means of interaction were completely inappropriate, not to mention unusable.

CASE STUDY OF DEBBIE F.

Other sections of this book explain in detail different individual techniques involved in the practice of phototherapy; my previous pages have dealt conceptually with the understandings necessary in working with clients who are somehow "different," and the people around them. I would like, therefore, to conclude with one case study as a more longitudinal example of the myriad possibilities available to therapists willing to interweave phototherapeutic techniques in their tapestry of helping skills. With this client, specific techniques were chosen, as all useful tools should be, when desired for specific purposes and goals, which I shall present along with their resultant effects. Although the main presenting disabling conditions were deafness and emotional/cultural deprivation, the techniques used are equally applicable to all physically/emotionally/culturally/societally handicapped or disadvantaged (as well as to the nondisabled or majority population!).

At the time we met, Debbie F. was a nine-year-old Native Indian girl who had been living in a Vancouver, B.C. (white) foster home since she had been brought down the coast at age three, because she had been diagnosed by her government social worker to be "deaf, emotionally disturbed, and in need of special medical care and education." She had already been through more pain and confusion than most adults ever have to face. As far as her family could tell, she had been born deaf, and her parents had no way of coping with the intricate consequences in their isolated small village. Badly burned in a house fire when she was two, Debbie had been in immediate need of numerous skin grafts and lengthy hospital confinements. Placed in a hospital several hundred miles from her village and her family, she had been required to stay there for many

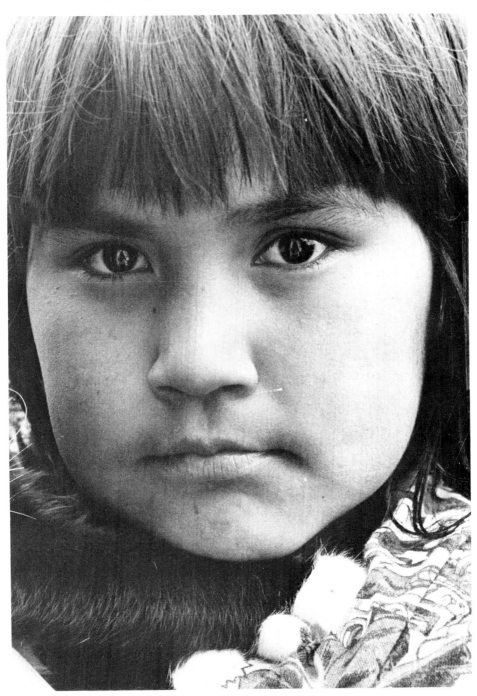

Copyright© 1980 by Judy Weiser

months — scared, confused, restrained in bed, and in severe pain; and unable, because of her deafness, to communicate anything with anyone, or be at all comforted by unfamiliar strangers.

Her mother's visits were very infrequent (at twenty, she had never before left her local area to go to a city), and Debbie's response on those occasions understandably was usually total rejection, brought on by her pain of perceived abandonment. The overall emotional trauma was so severe that Debbie would not trust or relate to anyone for years, and even today is extremely cautious with demonstrating her feelings or forming close relationships. As a child she was capable of only very basic primary verbal communication to express her slowly growing enthusiasm (which largely stayed locked inside), but with practice has been capable over her early teen years of large advances in her ability to communicate with the hearing culture in both nonverbal and verbal manners. This does not mean that she has become totally facile with the oral methods of lip-reading or speech production; nor does it mean she has abandoned her abilities to communicate in sign language — only that options have opened up for her over the many years of assistance, options that she did not even know existed when she first entered therapy. The general goals that have persisted over these years have been not to change her into something she is not (I have not sought to make a Native child white, or to make her "pass" as non-deaf), rather to make her more at home with herself as she is, and thus to be able to move more easily through the world around her.

Debbie is still a very emotionally complicated girl — in so many "marginal" statuses that she often becomes confused by their differing realities. She has had trouble with showing proper emotional affect in a situation, and often misreads the verbal and nonverbal cues that others give her. She has found it is difficult for people to understand her messages and their intent, and has long had trouble knowing how to fit into the world of those around her without standing out as "somehow different." The deaf/hearing consequences are fairly obvious; the Native Indian/white (even within a deaf group itself) is more subtle and harder to work out. These difficulties must be dealt with soon before late adolescence and adulthood complicate them further; she must somehow learn to become more comfortable and accepting of herself as well as presenting this to those around her.

Because of her increasing facility with speech and speech-reading, she is leaving the deaf "world" behind and trying to move into the hearing. This is being encouraged by her teachers who hope to "mainstream" her, and her foster mother who firmly believes that she is happier with hearing peers. This crossroads point gives those around her a rare opportunity to rigorously examine her perceptions for insight from the inside into the constructs of each different culture as viewed by this child with one foot on each side in several different situations. A better informant could rarely be found; but how to find it out?

In working with hearing-impaired children, especially pre-teens, one continually encounters kids who are feeling ideas, frustrations, and feelings that they *cannot* communicate to others, either because of disparities between sign language and English, or because (as with most children of any language) the very concepts causing concern just simply don't have enough subtle vocabulary developed yet to adequately label and explore these feelings.

Working with such children in therapy can be very frustrating and limiting for those whose styles are purely verbal/conversational. It simply will not do to ask such a child, "How did you feel when your Mommy never came to visit you?" Even if the child did somehow manage to understand the question itself (which, like most abstract concepts, is very difficult to learn to sign to younger deaf), she would probably find it extremely hard to try to convey those feelings (or even to reflect upon herself from an outside viewpoint enough to even recognize that she *has* those feelings).

With these kinds of clients I have frequently chosen to go about it photographically. In Debbie's case, armed with her simple Kodak and I with my 35 mm SLR (for camaraderie and comparisons of prints when desired), we have been going out exploring the world around Debbie, through *her* eyes and then through the examination of her prints. Sometimes we matched hers with mine of the same scene (such as scenery, people, animals — general random shots), which helped her to understand graphically the concepts I have been trying to get across to her abstractly because she was so affected by them; concepts such as selective perception, ethnocentrism and ego-centrism — the ways different people see the same thing differently and yet do not realize it, where there is no "right" or "wrong," only different. These things were very critical to this child who knew she was not like everyone else and spent much time trying to pursue the elusive "answer" that could make everything all right, who had no idea that she was worth just as much as the next person and that they were no more "right" than she was. These are things that I would have no way of telling her in any words or even in sign language, regardless of my fluency, because she simply could not at her age conceptualize that abstractly; even if she could, my words would have been disputable — with her own photos she could see for herself without any interference from me.

We went through numerous exercises geared for her showing me her world as she perceived it, and other exercises dealing with exploring specific topics that I chose to concentrate on because of their relevancy for therapy. For example, because of her relationship (or, rather, lack of it) with her mother, we spent a lot of time photographing women: women working, women "looking good," "happy" women, moving slowly to my target of more touchy assignments (to her) such as "good" mothers or mothers "being happy with their children" or mothers acting with their children as she though she might be with hers some-day, so that she could begin to explain to me (albeit indirectly) what she thought and how she felt about her mother's actions and how she interpreted them, and a way to defuse some of her hurt and anger by partializing the sub-ject into frozen moments of time in photos to examine her projections and selections and then to begin to interact with what she was seeing (and under-

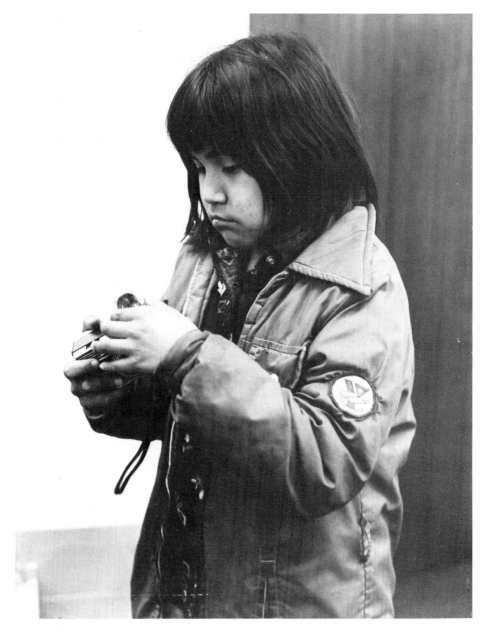

stand how and why she was seeing it that way). It was also a way to lead her toward future encounters with her mother (and photographing her mother — which definitely forms a relationship) that could be more healthily differentiated and open.

Another difficult area for Debbie was expressing and "reading" emotional affect. We studied what the idea of feelings meant and prepared several dozen such descriptive words on a list she wrote. The ones we decided were the most important of these (such as angry, happy, sad, mad, excited, uncertain, etc.) she wrote onto large index cards which we then worked with. Holding them under her chin, she would practice in a mirror, and then turn to me for a photo to be taken to document the "right" face. Alternatively she would take similar pictures of me or other children in her home doing the supposedly appropriate faces (although sometimes we might be testing her selection criteria by not always making the "right" faces). In later examining the prints to match faces and body postures to card labels, we were able to examine at arms length (and therefore less threateningly) how differently people see things and what one would have to do to portray a particular feeling in a particular situation in ways that other people would grasp the intent. Sometimes Debbie found she thought she was making one face, but the camera recorded it differently than she had expected. These exercises provided much room for safe dialogue and practice about things that she may have known about her inner self but could never have discussed in conversation. She was beginning to learn about herself, about her uniqueness and its value, about *how* she knew what she knew and made the value judgments she made.

One of the most potent techniques used with Debbie was the assignment of constructed albums when she was between eleven and thirteen. Family pressure had been mounting for her to have more contact with her village and her Native culture. Plans were made for her to start spending her summers up north, where basically no one really knew her or how to communicate with her (and where she had not been since a small child). She was extremely ambivalent — wanting to "meet" her real parents, and yet very anxious and afraid, and worried that they might not let her return to her foster mother (and also that the other village children would be shy and judgmental and not play with her). She was not sure what they would be expecting of her or how to find it out. And, once there, she would have no further contact with the "outside world" until the return trip to Vancouver. It promised to be a very long summer, and she had to be as prepared as possible to cope with almost anything. As winter progressed, her school chums, resenting all the attention she was receiving, had begun to tease her about anything that would goad a response — the strongest of which was that she was an "unwanted" child, that she had really been found in a garbage can and did not have any real parents. As a solution to all of these complexities, I decided Debbie should make two photo albums over the spring and summer months: a "Vancouver" book to take north with her, and a "Village" book of photos to bring back to describe her experiences while there. We spent time discussing what things about her life in the city were important to her and that she would want to show the people up north so they could see who she was. Lists were also made of the things she knew she would want to take pictures of once in her village--such as her parents, brothers and sister,

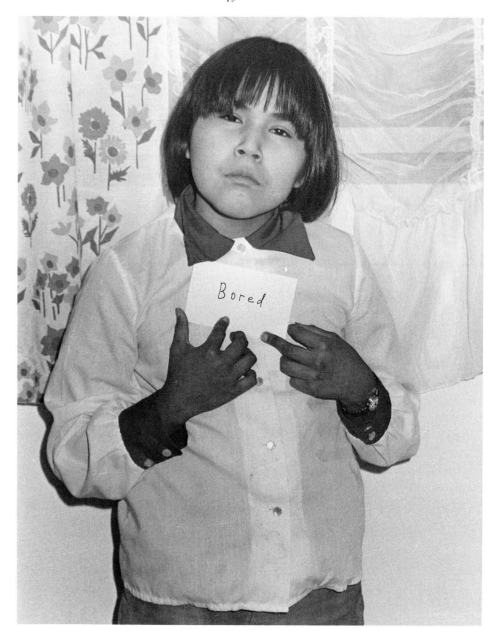

their home, the school, church, store, etc. She spent many weeks photographing the topics on the first list, chose her own favorites, and put the album together by herself — it was *her* book organized (and spelled!) in her own unique way; no teacher was going to demand any corrections or changes, and she greatly enjoyed that. The first album, finished in time for her to take with

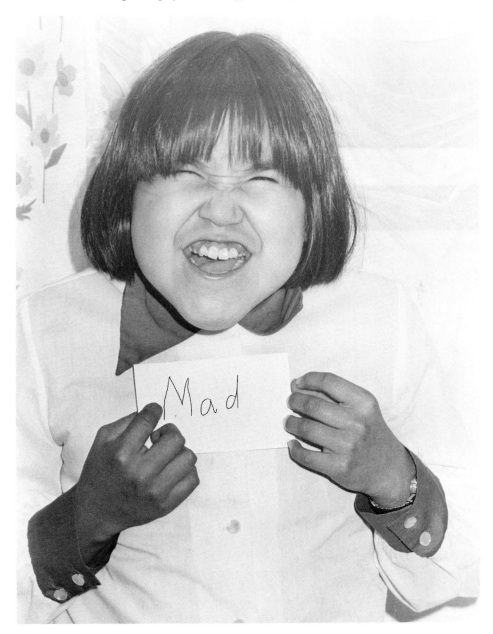

her on her journey north included pages on "my house," "my room," "my cats," "trips to other places," "my friends," "school," "Christmas and the tree and presents," "silly people," etc., i.e. the differences that made a difference in her life at that time.

Showing the book to family and neighbors once she had arrived in the

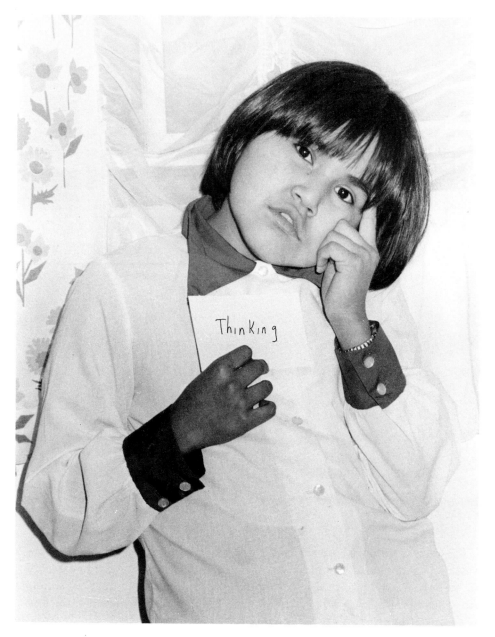

village, Debbie could point to parallels as a communication tool (point to foster mom and then her own mother, her brother's bike he sat upon, and then her bike in the photo, and then herself, etc.). People were not so hesitant or frightened of her as she was more approachable through a means of communication, tensions relaxed as a form of "charades" developed with the help of the album. She appeared normal — she had a scrapbook just like other people had; she did not have to sit invisibly in a group of people who wanted to meet her but did not know how. And an additional result was that her family was able to gain some idea of what her life in the city was actually like on a day-to-day basis (and thus coming to visit her there did not seem like such an alien experience to be worried about, did not seem all that different on a daily basis from life in the village — and in fact reassured her parents of her being well taken care of). When her parents had the opportunity to visit the city the following winter, her surroundings did not seem so foreign, as they had seen them before, and they had time to know what to expect.

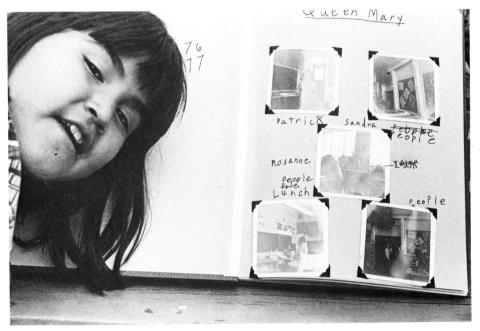

Copyright© 1980 by Judy Weiser

The second album, to be recorded while up north, proved to be more interesting in its creation. . . Armed with her second list of "what to photograph" that summer in the village, as well as an ample supply of film for her simple auto-set camera, Debbie arrived for her visit. I accompanied her in for the first day's transition as she was still too young to travel alone, and met her family. I took a few rolls of my own slide film for general interest (including Debbie with her parents, their home, etc.), and then left. At the end of the summer, I anxiously awaited her return (and photos) — only to find that she'd lost her camera overboard the second day out on her dad's fishboat, and thus had lots of film (unexposed) but no camera. I suppose one should pause here for some sort of existential comment about therapists maintaining a sense of humor and not taking ourselves too seriously in this profession. . .The problem

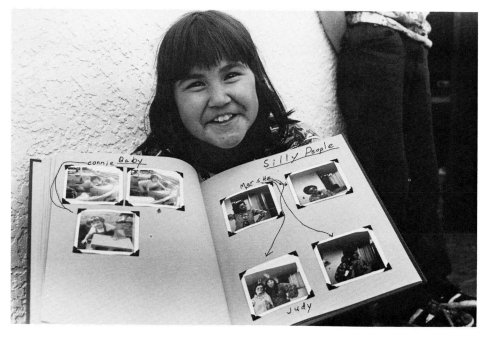

Copyright© 1980 by Judy Weiser

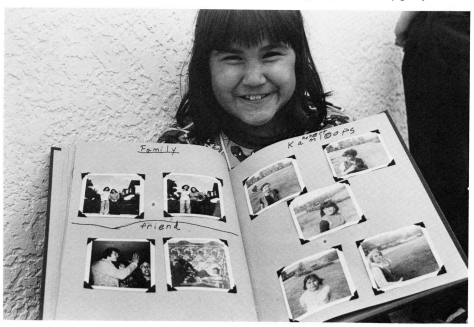

Copyright© 1980 by Judy Weiser

was mostly solved, however, by converting my slides into prints for her book, which she then proudly took to school to show her classmates. Once one has seen the photos of her with her parents there is no doubt of her lineage; they

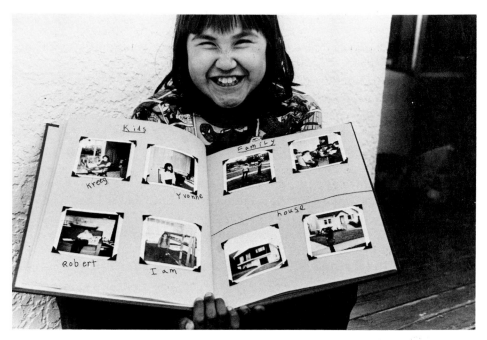

look identical!

Less direct but still powerful benefits came from this album work. Debbie came back with a tangible identity that she could refer back to at any time and show to people who never before could comprehend her past or her family relationships. She began to tie together her present life with her roots. Her snapshots offered frozen moments with her family which she could study, in amounts she could handle (and in privacy), what she thought about them and her relationship to them, as well as beginning to outwardly share her thoughts and feelings because she had time to put it all in order. She began to comprehend places existing simultaneously in time and what her position is in relation to each. Making the section on "a typical week in winter in Vancouver" helped her to better grasp time and continuity concepts, and she began to manage more comfortably concepts of regular dependable cycles of time and actions/consequences. The easier the ties between past/present/future became, the less frightened she was of getting lost between them, and the less anxious of losing her identity to the void.

Having shared some experiences in common while showing her album and comparing lives with her family gave all of them some subject material and memories to begin written communication in between visits, and the depersonalized barriers began to fall as the two "worlds" began to be bridged. But best of all the albums gave Debbie more of a grasp on who she is, and a sense of self-worth both in the making of them and in their contents, and additionally she was able to begin to see her own part in things, her own responsibilities in and ties to the process of events. She became better able to change the parts of herself she was dissatisfied with by analyzing them and their implications to her life.

New experiences and people continued to be added to the album collection, and we also began a special section on "moods" whereby she could add to any page an indication of her feelings toward each photograph. It interested her (and taught her as well) to realize these continually were changing. We went a step further into rewarding her curiosities with lessons in darkroom techniques, because I had become increasingly aware over the years that this young lady had artistic talent beyond our therapeutic exercises. She was very quick to pick up the basics of printing (she most definitely is *not* retarded, as I had first been told), and has continued for many years her interest and practice in the darkroom. There have been many therapeutic benefits to this as well, as in the first day she voluntarily printed and chose to keep a portrait of her mother that she had taken on a visit, or discussions around why she decided to "crop out" her brother from a family picture. Her pride in her new skills was evident. The added confidence spread to her school tasks, and she began to better understand more abstract concepts such as delayed gratification and cause/effect/responsibility-for-consequence, once she had been through them tangibly yet simply in the darkroom.

Debbie has grown to be better centered, and has gained constructive outlets for her emotions, better able to hold onto her multicontexts without as much confusion. These few examples above are all special lessons in two-way interactive communication, an attempt to notice cultural consensus or differences as to what is being expressed, and how to notice it "correctly." They are ways to learn how another person perceives and judges. If the photographs taken show "cultural errors" in perception or interpretation, these can be noted and discussed. A person of any age will be much less defensive discussing a neutral object such as a photograph, while leaving themselves somewhat protected until feeling comfortable enough to be a bit more vulnerable in discussing more personal things. Similarly, in work with Debbie, it is clear that she has begun to feel for the first time in her life that communication with the hearing world and also the white world is within her grasp, and that although it may not be in a totally verbal fashion, that she now has alternatives to fall back upon to make her thoughts and feelings known to others (and herself). Debbie "fits" better these days.

CLOSURE. . .
CAMERAS DON'T TAKE PICTURES; PEOPLE DO!

Hopefully the previous pages have provided the theoretical rationale and many practical techniques for implementing the use of photography as a tool in

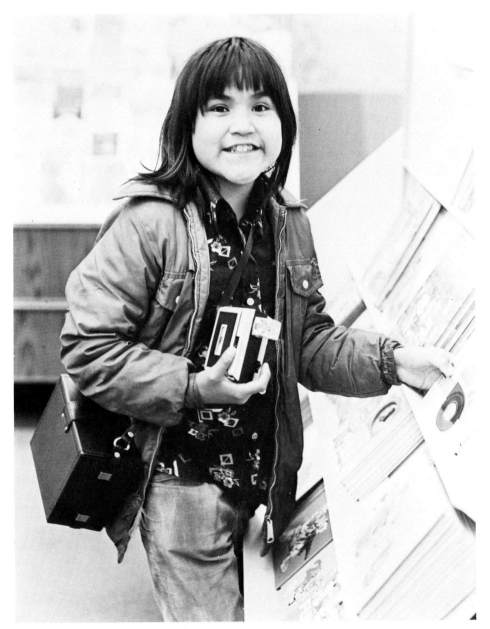

assisting the process of growth and change for clients, including those who are physically, emotionally or culturally disabled or disadvantaged (both the individual and those around them). As long as photography remains as important to our society as it is now, phototherapy will not be just another "fad" therapy. The use and understanding of the photographic image is central to our visual literacy, and the use of that literacy will expand further within the scope of therapeutic relationships (Stewart, 1979).

It is essential that better training be provided for therapists to learn to appropriately use these techniques, to learn to fully "read" photographs, to know how to ask the proper questions and how to deal with the information that emerges, to fine tune one's attention to the photograph and the process involved in exploring it, as well as the ability to point out to the client on what data the observations are based. Special skill in photography itself is unnecessary, but further training in the visual and/or metaphoric modes is essential. It must be stressed that there are no "phototherap*ists*," per se, and that each competent therapist uses a unique combination of helping skills and knows which tools to use for the presenting situation; phototherapeutic techniques are invaluable additions to these collections of "what to do," but it is not intended that the therapist exclude all other potentially helpful possibilities. Phototherapy is not some kind of "voodoo"; there is no special secret mysterious skill involved. It just takes training, practice, and an open curious mind — and a commitment to work within the value system of the client rather than interpreting meaning for them (as well as trying to keep the therapist's own personal agenda out of it all!).

. . . .

DONNA IN THERAPY

Donna in therapy
Shows me a picture:
Two people stand
In a park,
A lake beyond,
Bushes beside.

           She,

The woman crisp
In worldwar skirt,

           he,

The man in shirtsleeves
Rolled toward the elbow,
Arm around her,

           pulling

But she's firm.

           He bends

From the ground--
Sapling twisted
Toward the sun.

           This

Is my mother,
She said firmly.

Copyright© 1979
Arnold Gassan

One must learn and then practice the concept that there is no "right" and "wrong" in this business — only "different," and that the therapist as well as the client can learn to expect, understand, and appreciate the differences and differentness. Photography is a powerful medium. "Everyone has seen photographs that *really* shook them up. Some things you see are just almost too much to bear. That power is available to damn near anybody. You know it's available to you; it's available to me; you just have to figure it out" (Hattersley, 1980).

REFERENCES

Bandler, R. and Grinder, J. *Frogs into princes.* Palo Alto, CA: Science and Behavior Books, 1979.

Chinn, P.C., Winn, J., and Walters, R. *Two-way talking with parents of special children.* St. Louis, MO: C.V. Mosby Co., 1978.

Freeman, R.D. Assessment and treatment of a family with a disabled member. Paper presented at the Fifth Western Canadian Conference on Family Practice, May, 1981.

Gassan, A. Collection of Poems. Private publication; personal communication, 1979.

Hattersley, R. Thirty ways photography is good for you. *Popular Photography,* 1980, February, 87-127.

Krauss, D. Photography, imaging, and visually referent language in therapy: Illuminating the metaphor. *Camera Lucida,* 1981, *5.*

Kübler-Ross, E. *Death — the final stage of growth.* Englewood Cliffs, NJ: Prentice-Hall, 1975.

Stewart, D. Photography comes of age. *Kansas Quarterly,* 1979, 2(4).

Turner-Hogan, P. The use of group photo therapy in the classroom. *Photo Therapy Quarterly,* 1981, *2(4),* 13.

Note: A full bibliography of over 500 sources (background readings and specific references) can be ordered from the author. Judy Weiser, 1107 Homer, 3rd Floor, Vancouver BC, CANADA V6B 2Y2.

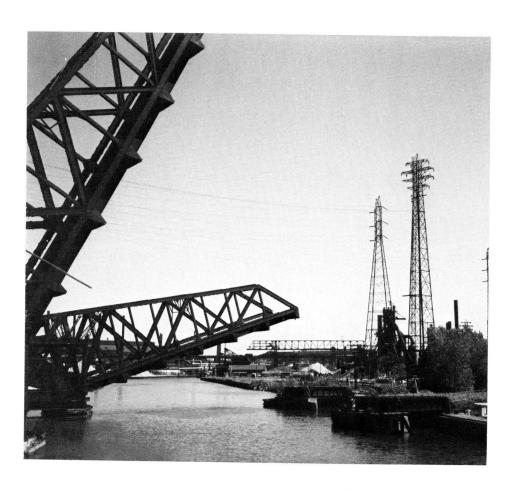

Photo by David A. Krauss

Chapter 11

Phototherapy Intervention: Developing a Comprehensive System

BRIAN ZAKEM

INTRODUCTION

THE first relationship between photography and professional mental health services was documented in 1852, when psychiatrist Diamond reported using still phototherapy interventions with his chronic, institutionalized patients (Gilman, 1976). This followed by just thirteen years the public announcement of the invention of photography in 1839. It took more than 100 years following Diamond's pioneering work for a comprehensive system of phototherapy interventions to begin to be formulated (Zakem, 1978, 1979; Stewart, 1979 a,b, 1980). Phototherapy interventions have expanded to include motion pictures (Rothschild, 1979) and video recordings (Muzekari, 1975; Berger, 1978; Fryrear and Fleshman, 1981), with implications for holographic images.

Until recently, the literature on phototherapy primarily consisted of anecdotal case reports; clinical research and practice studies which often lacked scientific rigor and/or the knowledge of previous relevant literature in phototherapy; and descriptive articles about phototherapy interventions (Loellbach, 1978). On the whole, the most recent literature has reflected greater attention to scientific rigor and knowledge of the relevant literature base, e.g. Krauss, 1979; Stewart, 1980; Hall, 1981. Fortunately, as the scientifically "maturing" phototherapy literature overcomes these earlier shortcomings, a richer dialogue between practice and research is fostered. This, in turn, promotes the development of more reliable and replicable phototherapy interventions (Metcoff, 1980).

A major goal of the cooperative work between phototherapy practitioners and researchers is the development of a comprehensive system of phototherapy intervention. By a comprehensive system, this writer is referring to the incorporation of contemporary photography options into a systematic treatment of service delivery plan. Such a system is based upon the "state of the art" of relevant social-psychological and behavioral sciences, as well as on mental health and phototherapy intervention research, integrated with effective clinical practice skills. Such a comprehensive system must eventually elucidate the elements of phototherapy interventions that tend to produce reliable and effective results. Hopefully these efforts will lead to the scientific demonstration of effective interventions as well as the delineation of mental health intervention variables that tend to increase the probability of desirable treatment outcomes (Strupp, 1978).

Orlinsky and Howard's (1978) definition of "psychotherapy" encompasses all components of the framework being proposed for developing a comprehensive system of phototherapy interventions. They define psychotherapy as

> (1) a relation among persons, engaged in by (2) one or more individuals defined as needing special assistance to (3) improve their functioning as persons, together with (4) one or more individuals defined as able to render such special help. (p. 284)

The first part of their definition deals with the relationship process in all-encompassing terms; the second and fourth parts refer to the specific minimal conditions required to participate in mental health interventions; and the third part suggests the terms that deal with the outcomes. This definition does not exclude ". . . any of the specific practices, findings and perspectives that have been significant in clinical [mental health] work" (Orlinsky and Howard, p. 283); thus, it is compatible with phototherapy's contemporary, multidisciplinary orientation.

A FRAMEWORK FOR DEVELOPING A COMPREHENSIVE SYSTEM OF PHOTOTHERAPY INTERVENTION

The outline below consists of three sections, organized to provide a framework for developing a comprehensive system of phototherapy intervention. Section I is a classification of the basic mental health service components (Subsection A based on Korchin, 1976; Subsection B based on Corsini, 1973). Section II (based on Metcoff, 1980) lists and describes the basic components considered necessary in the planning and implementing stages of a well-designed phototherapy intervention. Section III is a listing of contemporary photography options and variations available to client and therapist or change agent, which can be effectively integrated into phototherapy interventions. These options can be used singly or in combination.

Recent advances in the technology of photography have led to the ability to transfer images between stills, motion pictures, and video recordings.

I. *Mental Health Service Components*
A. Clinical and/or Field Assessment
    1. To understand the individual(s) personality and functioning from each of these six basic perspectives:
       a. motivational
       b. structural
       c. developmental
       d. adaptational

    e. ecological

    f. biological

  2. By means of:

    a. informal techniques, i.e. structured and nonstructured interviews and observations

    b. formal techniques, i.e. standardized individual and group testing, including projective and psychometric personality, intelligence, vocational tests, etc., as well as neuropsychological and neuropsychiatric tests for psychosomatic and/or organic/chemical originated disorders

B. Contemporary Psychological and Organic Therapies

  1. Psychological major orientations

    a. analytic

    b. behavioral

    c. humanistic-existential

    d. eclectic

  2. Psychiatric major orientation is psychopharmacology

C. Modalities of Mental Health Service

  1. individual

  2. couple

  3. family

  4. group

  5. milieu

  6. community

  7. organization or institution

D. Training Professionals, Paraprofessionals, and Lay Persons

  1. formal academic work

  2. formal clinical internships and practica

  3. clinical supervision

  4. continuing education, i.e. didactic and experiential

  5. professionally run and supervised clinical experiences, and continuing education opportunities for competency in these mental health service roles

E. Research

  1. scientific studies in clinic, field or lab setting

  2. communication of findings to the allied mental health professions, as well as clear translation into lay terms for clients, potential consumers, and other interested persons

  3. feedback to mental health researchers from clinicians and clients concerning the effects of applied mental health sciences.

II. *Basic Components of Phototherapy Intervention*

A. Goal(s)

  1. diagnostic evaluation designed to determine goal(s) in relationship

to the assessed problems of the client(s)

2. Determine plan of intervention, designed to effectively aid client in attaining goal(s), measurable by indicators of emotional, behavioral and/or physiological changes

3. Implement intervention(s), which can be conceptualized within one or more of the following categories (based on Fryrear, 1980):
   a. self-confrontation
   b. evoking emotional states
   c. eliciting verbal behavior
   d. modeling
   e. aiding socialization experiences
   f. self-expression and creativity
   g. photo images as nonverbal communication from client to therapist or change agent, or vice versa
   h. documentation of physical change
   i. mastery of a skill, improving self-esteem
   j. therapeutic usefulness of "keepsake" photos at termination

4. Evaluate interventions

B. Appropriate Timing

   At what phase of an intervention, or stage of therapy or consultation does the therapist or change agent introduce selected phototherapy techniques, depending on treatment plan and goals?

C. Arrangement of Photographic Materials

1. How does the therapist or change agent introduce materials to the client?

2. What effect(s) on the client does the presence and arrangement of material(s) have?

3. What are the rules, stated and implied, of integrating the materials into the client/therapist or change agent relationship?

D. Role of Therapist or Change Agent

1. When appropriate, the therapist or change agent aids the focus of attention and dialogue with the client regarding photographic materials and helps establish therapy goals

2. Supports or directs decisions concerning how to use these materials, which of these materials to use, view, or review, when and by whom

3. Aids in evaluating the phototherapy experience with the client

4. Aids the client's integration of emotional, behavioral, and/or physiological change with intervention and life-style

E. Viewing and Reviewing Effects of Photo Images

1. Known responses to the presentation of photographic images, including increased interest in self-image, recall of content, attention span, and learning about behaviors of self and others, etc. are used

by the therapist or change agent to aid the goal(s) of intervention
  F. Target Audience for the Phototherapy Intervention
      1. Who is going to see the images selected and/or produced?
      2. To aid what goal(s)?
  III. *Contemporary Photography Options*
  A. Still(s)
      1. Instant prints from instant developing film and photograms
      2. Darkroom processed prints and slide transparencies
  B. Motion Pictures
      1. Instant movies from instant developing movie film
      2. Darkroom processed movies (with or without special effects).
  C. Videotape/Videodisc Recordings
      1. Instant recording from magnetic tape or disc
      2. In the forms of silent or sound, and black and white or color, with or without special effects (such as computer graphics), still frame, slow, actual, and fast motion
  D. Holographic Images (based on Dowbenko, 1978)
      1. Wet processed stills, three-dimensional visual representation
        a. transmission
        b. reflection
      2. Instant processed stills
      3. Wet processed, multiplex motion, 360° images
      4. In the forms of silent or sound, and black and white or color, with or without special effects, still frame, slow, actual, and fast motion

A CLINICAL APPLICATION OF THE FRAMEWORK

A clinical application of the framework, illustrating how it can aid the planning and implementation of an appropriately designed phototherapy intervention, follows.

The process of planning and implementing any effective mental health intervention begins at intake. At this point, a clinical assessment of each client is made, based upon psychological, psychiatric, and medical findings derived from interviews, observation, examinations, and, as indicated, psychological and medical tests. In this illustration, the entire Adult Psychiatric Day Hospital staff of Ravenswood Hospital Community Mental Health Center reviews these reports, together with any additional referral information, at a clinical meeting, and makes a determination of the client's appropriateness for the Day Hospital program. If the client is accepted, the primary therapist formulates an individual intervention plan based upon this review of the data. The staff designs specific milieu interventions to respond to the problems that the client group is experiencing in common. These interventions are designed to complement other modalities of service each client is receiving, such as individual, family, and group therapy.

Twenty clients, ranging in age from twenty to sixty-five years, comprised the Day Hospital client group in November, 1978, when this phototherapy intervention was introduced. As a group, they could accurately be described as being acutely or chronically depressed, although the severity of their underlying disorders and their diagnoses varied. The behavior of these clients tended to be passive, resulting in social and emotional isolation from one another. This isolation was often reflected in their relationships with their families, friends, and acquaintances.

Given this background data, the staff decided to introduce a series of weekly phototherapy interventions, the goal of which was to aid socialization experiences. Indicators of goal attainment included reduction of depressive signs, such as an increase in activity level. This intervention would be congruent with other Day Hospital interventions, and would support the program's mission of building a cohesive, supportive milieu.

The staff began designing methods and procedures to aid in the attainment of the stated goal. We thought that an experience based on voluntary participation would minimize resistance, and that an intervention spanning several weekly sessions, rather than being completed during a single session, would be more effective. The staff also decided to try to build fun into the experience. The outcome of these considerations was to design a sound movie project, to be completed within a single two-hour session. The participants included the twenty clients, two staff, and three graduate student clinicians.

We were aware that some clients might find this activity too self-confronting and anxiety-producing for their fragile personality structure. In an effort to reduce fears and anxiety, the activity was structured so as to provide clients with options relating to their degree and type of participation. The persons involved could choose to participate either in making the movie or in documenting that process. The documentary options included the choice of participating as a member of either the instant still photography group or the videotape recording group. By offering these options, we hoped that the clients would make their selection based on their level of comfort with the project tasks.

Since we hoped to maintain interest in this intervention over a period of several weeks, we wanted to create photographic products that could be viewed and reviewed with continuing interest. By working with the photographic products generated during this intervention, the staff also hoped to aid the attainment of other secondary intervention goals, such as eliciting verbal behavior, documenting physical changes that occurred during this intervention, and mastering a skill, thus improving self-esteem. In general, the staff expected this intervention to facilitate the process of developing a more cohesive, supportive, and active client group.

In addition to being given complete freedom to choose among the three photographic options to engage in, the participants could further negotiate a specific role for themselves with the other members of their selected task group. They could also switch from one group to another if they so chose. We hoped that by offering these options, we would maximize participation and encourage people to enter into the project in whatever manner they felt most comfortable. In fact, everyone agreed to participate in the initial intervention, and almost all continued to participate during the following weekly sessions.

The formal phototherapy intervention began by assembling the clients and participating staff and students, and presenting them with a semi-structured task; specifically, to produce a three and one-half minute color sound movie of their choice. Prior to this, the staff and students had arranged the photographic equipment, film, and videotapes alongside the large hospital room within which the intervention would take place. The rationale for this arrangement was to allow easy access to the equipment and materials without suggesting how the participants might choose to use them. This arrangement was designed to encourage the use of all three photographic options, without singling out any one option as being more valued by staff and students. The two staff members stood by as technical consultants simply to explain the operation of the equipment, without communicating their preference. In addition, they did not select a group task to participate in until all of the clients had made their initial selection.

The movie makers formed a group of 10 members, while two smaller groups, of five members each, formed to document this process. It was noted that the movie production group appeared to be the most active, and was mostly comprised of the more active female members of the milieu. They quickly assigned leadership roles to direct and produce the film, and began shooting the movie within an hour. In contrast, the still photo documentary group, comprised mostly of middle aged, passive males, was less active, although they did begin to take several rolls of film of the work of the other two groups within the first hour. The activity level of the videotape recording group, comprised mostly of young, single males, was comparable to the still film group.

The film was completed shortly after the first hour. Since it was not instant film, the viewing of the processed movie would take place the following week. In the meantime, the entire group could begin to view and review the stills and video documentation. The still photos were displayed in the order taken, and people were encouraged to share their perceptions of the photos individually and in sequence.

After this process was completed, the author asked for a volunteer who had actually been in the movie to rearrange the photos in the order she perceived the movie to have taken place. Of interest, the volunteer reorganized the sequential ordering of the photos. Her personal perspective of the events that had occurred just an hour earlier and her perception of the content of some of the photos were reasonable. This led to further discussion of different perspectives of this event. The videotape recording and processed movie awaited viewing and reviewing by the group as a whole in the ensuing weeks.

This weekly series of phototherapy interventions significantly increased the frequency and quality of socialization of this client group, as confirmed by staff and client observation over the next several weeks.

Conclusion

The work that needs to be undertaken to ensure the maturation of a comprehensive system of mental health interventions parallels the needs of a comprehensive system of phototherapy interventions. Both require that a dialogue be fostered between mental health practitioners and researchers in order to generate useful research and evalution of phototherapy interventions. This ongoing communication and feedback will help answer such questions as

- How do phototherapy interventions actually work to effect certain processes or outcomes?
- How effective are specific phototherapy interventions compared to other mental health interventions?
- What effect(s) do specific components of phototherapy interventions have, with which individuals, and with which behavior/personality dimensions?
- How can phototherapy be incorporated into a comprehensive treatment plan, and to meet which client needs?

The mental health sciences lack clear, empirical evidence of how specific intervention variables interact to effect successful outcomes in clients with specific psychological problems. Thus, it is imperative that we begin to ". . . set up good, empirical research projects in order to make efficacy claims of procedures" (Garfield and Bergin, 1978, p. ix), and to investigate the " . . . effectiveness of therapeutic procedures, as well as therapists . . . by systematic research" (Garfield and Bergin, p. ix).

The recent trends in phototherapy interventions are in the direction of developing a more systematic, comprehensive and scientifically based system. More knowledgeable planning, design, and implementation of specific phototherapy techniques will necessarily lead to higher standards of professional accountability.

A word of caution. Although phototherapy has recently attained a systematic, rigorous scientific orientation, it is important that practitioners and researchers do not prematurely overstate its effectiveness. The framework presented in this chapter is an attempt to facilitate the ongoing development of a more scientifically based system of phototherapy intervention.

REFERENCES

Berger, M. (Ed.), *Videotape techniques in psychiatric training and treatment, 2nd. Ed.* New York: Brunner/Mazel, 1978.

Corsini, R. (Ed.), *Current psychotherapies.* Itasca, IL.: F.E. Peacock, 1-73.

Dowbenko, G. *Homegrown holography.* Garden City, N.Y.: Amphoto, 1978.

Fryrear, J.L. A selective non-evaluative review of research on phototherapy. *Phototherapy, 2*(3), 1981, 7-9.

Fryrear, J.L., and Fleshman, R. (Eds.) *Videotherapy in mental health.* Springfield, IL.: Charles C Thomas, Publisher, 1981.

Garfield, S., and Bergin, A. The handbook of psychotherapy and behavior change. New York: John Wiley and Sons, 1978.

Gilman, S. (Ed.), *The face of madness.* New York: Brunner/Mazel, 1976.

Hall, D. Photography as a learning experience in self-perception. Doctoral Dissertation, University of Michigan, 1981.

Korchin, S. *Modern clinical psychology.* New York: Basic Books, 1976.

Krauss, D.A The uses of still photography in counseling and therapy: Development of a training model. Doctoral Dissertation, Kent State University, 1979.

Loellbach, M. The uses of photographic materials in psychotherapy: A literature review. *Phototherapy* publication reprints, Houston, TX, 1978.

Metcoff, J. Towards a pragmatic description of a video intervention. *Phototherapy, 2*(3), 1980, 4-7.

Muzekari, L. An annotated bibliography on the use of television and videotape in treatment and research. Behavioral Science Clinical Research Center, Philadelphia State Hospital, 1975. Unpublished.

Orlinsky, D., and Howard, K. The relation of process to outcome in psychotherapy. In S. Garfield and A. Bergin (Eds.) *The handbook of psychotherapy and behavior change.* New York: John Wiley and Sons, 1978.

Rothschild, J. Phototherapy: Film animation as a therapeutic tool. Master's study, Illinois Institute of Technology, 1979.

Stewart, D. Phototherapy comes of age. *Kansas Quarterly, 2* (4), 1979, 19-46. (a)

Stewart, D. Phototherapy: Theory and practice. *Art Psychotherapy, 6*(1), 1979, 41-46. (b)

Stewart, D. The use of client photographs as self statements in phototherapy. Doctoral Dissertation, Northern Illinois University, 1980.

Strupp, H. Psychotherapy research and practice: An overview. In S. Garfield and A. Bergin (Eds.), *The handbook of pyschotherapy and behavior change.* New York: John Wiley and Sons, 1978.

Zakem, B. Definition of phototherapy's range and scope. *Phototherapy, 1*(2), 1978, 1.

Zakem, B. Editorial. *Phototherapy, 2*(1), 1979, 1-2.

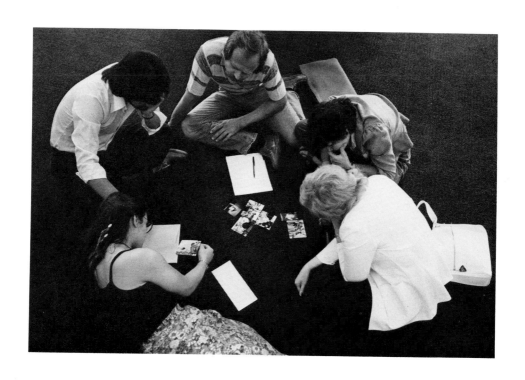

Photo by David A. Krauss

Chapter 12

A Training Model for the Use of Still Photography in Therapy

DAVID A. KRAUSS AND ANSEL L. WOLDT

We think of teaching as a process by which teacher and students create a shared environment including sets of values and beliefs (agreements about what is important) which in turn color their view of reality. The "models" of teaching which are chosen to pattern teaching activities have much to say about the kinds of realities which will be admitted to the classroom and the kinds of life-view which are likely to be generated as teacher and learner work together. (Joyce & Weil, 1972, p. 3)

APPLIED phototherapy encompasses a myriad of techniques that are constantly being invented, adapted and refined by mental health practitioners. These techniques include a vast array of useful interventions that range from enhancing normal youngsters' self-esteem by teaching them the craft of photography and the subsequent open-ended discussion of their work, to assessing schizophrenics' reality contact by taking their picture and having subsequent discussion. Most interventions use photographs from the past; photographs of clients made by self or others, or photographs of others. Photographs can be used as a way of making contact, collecting information, teaching a skill, learning a point of view, creating projections, shaping behavior and enhancing self-concept. Surprisingly, very little skill is needed by the practitioner in the craft of photography itself to work in the modality. Sufficient skills can be acquired with a "point and shoot" conventional or an instant camera in a matter of minutes.

This chapter presents an example of a training model of phototherapy. Teaching the craft of photography is beyond the scope of this chapter; however there are a number of books on the topic mentioned in the references for this book by Gasson, Hattersley, Muse, and Swedlung. The phototherapist may be particularly interested in Gasson's *Handbook for Contemporary Photography* because it not only is a fine introductory photography text but also because it deals with the concept of "meaning" in photographs. The Hattersley book *Discover Yourself Through Photography* contains a number of exercises that may not only be self-instructive but also suggest phototherapy techniques that may be used as client homework assignments.

211

To simply list or teach all existing phototherapy techniques would not only be impossible, given the dynamic and fluent nature of these practices, it would also be inconsistent with the nature of therapeutic interventions as they are always situation specific. The use of any intervention calls for the proper assessment of a number of variables such as level of trust, readiness for change, willingness to risk, proper timing, and so forth, all of which are mediated by the therapist's style. Krauss's research (1979) demonstrated that phototherapy can be taught and this chapter systematically examines several major topic areas in which photography has been used as a therapeutic adjunct with clients. For purposes of training we have divided these areas into their most distinct attributes (such as self-portraits or projections); however, it should be clear there is much overlap in actual practice. The principles found in these topic areas can be used to enhance clinicians' intervention strategies and their ability to model and respond to clients with more appropriate, creative, and divergent behavior, thus helping their clients to see their therapy differently, enhancing insight and providing outlook that allows them to see their problems and potential solutions more clearly.

In training mental health professionals to be able to use photography in their work with clients, the authors have a number of beliefs, concerns, and expectations. We believe that although most clinicians have been trained in verbal modalities of counseling and therapy, few have had much training utilizing the visual modality. We are concerned that a valid, expanded repertoire of skills be learned so that client needs may be more fully met in counseling and therapy. Phototherapy fits well into this enlarged perspective of training because of the dominant visual and/or nonverbal orientation of some clients as they experience the world around them. Hence, photographs can serve as metaphors of a client's reality; they show how a client sees the world.

Photographs are also well suited to counseling and therapy sessions as they provide a vast amount of information about a client's history and life-style that can lead quickly to meaningful dialogue between client and practitioner. Photographs allow a professional to enter the client's world, see that world through his/her eyes, learn the vocabulary and syntax of that world and help the client to change his/her vocabulary and perception. In this way, a practitioner shows a client different options for viewing and experiencing his/her life.

In teaching this theoretical approach and its applied techniques, the authors believe it is important to create a curriculum that "instructs" (facilitates learning) on both the professional and personal level and that engages both cognitive and affective aspects of the learner. We seek to influence students to use phototherapy in flexible ways with their clients, in ways that best serve client needs. Once the techniques of phototherapy are demonstrated, they are seen almost immediately as useful tools for the profession; however, their integrated use by practitioners comes about much more readily and fully as a result of their own personal experience with the techniques.

The use of learner photographs in the teaching model is crucial. It is from viewing, discussing, and working with participants' personal photographs that the true power, validity, and elegance of this approach become apparent. In personalizing the phototherapy training in this manner, two other theoretical (or value) statements are also made. The first is that it is important for all mental health practitioners to be aware of and work on their own needs and concerns in life. In doing this kind of self house-cleaning, clinicians are less likely to confuse their own themes with those of their clients so that in therapy the focus is on client rather than therapist issues. Secondly, these techniques, like all interventions, should be used when it is the clinician's opinion that this particular intervention might be the most helpful for the client now, and that this judgment is derived from the experience of the therapeutic relationship. No technique is a substitute for contact with a client. Without the proper context of contact, trust, and timing, all techniques are mere exercises — dry, empty, and lifeless. The above values are stated and modeled during the phototherapy training sessions.

It is important in advertising the workshops and in the first training session, to provide participants with a clear understanding and agreement that part of the learning process involves their personal participation in the techniques to be studied. The program, therefore, contains components for both personal and professional awareness, insight, and growth.

In the numerous workshops we have conducted/taught at Kent State University, a wide range of professionals and paraprofessionals have participated in our training. Participants have included psychologists, counselors, psychiatrists, social workers, teachers, administrators, school psychologists, artists, art therapists, photographers, media specialists, a headmistress, nurses, a director of day treatment program, a group home manager and various professors of visual arts, psychology and psychiatry. Having a broad represenation from these many helping professions has contributed to the learning environment and broadened the spectrum of applications of phototherapy beyond those commonly considered within more narrowly focused professions. Interestingly, these widely divergent training groups have enthusiastically merged their creative energies through the phototherapy processes and unanimously endorsed the continued training of professionals in this medium.

This training orientation is a synthesis of the authors' learnings about learning as educators and psychotherapists. We have, in part, combined theories of group investigation, as proposed by Herbert Thelen (1960); laboratory method, as developed at the National Training Laboratory in Bethel, Maine; awarenss training, as written about by Schutz (1967), confluent education, as written about by Brown (1971, 1975) and gestalt therapy as developed by Perls (1951) and his numerous followers such as Polster and Polster (1973).

Instructional Equipment

In class, Polaroid and Kodak Instant print cameras, as well as Instamatic-type cameras can be utilized by students, as the focus of this course is on phototherapy techniques and not photographic skills per se. This equipment is preferred because it is relatively inexpensive, it can be operated by almost anyone with minimal instruction, it is generally available to the public, and because it can be readily employed in the practice setting.

The classroom itself might well be equipped with a videotape camera, recorder and large monitor, as well as a slide projector. This equipment can be used as teaching aids, as well as tools to gather data about the class. The video camera and monitor, for example, can be utilized to effectively facilitate the enlargement of a small photo or snapshot so that the entire class can view it simultaneously on the monitor screen. It is well to have a slide projector and screen available for participants who choose that type of photo.

We suggest that evaluation be a two-way process variable to be incorporated throughout the training, rather than a static type of final examination. For example, we believe it is important to have participants demonstrate their ability to formulate questions and observations based on the data contained in photographs, and to receive feedback instantly from others regarding their ability. In a final assessment of the workshop is desired, we suggest the use of sentence completion items, and to consider the use of sentence stubs such as:

> "I most liked. . . . .
> "I least liked. . . . .
> "I'd change. . . . .
> "I'd appreciate more. . . . .
> "In phototherapy I am best at. . . . .
> "In my continued professional development as phototherapist, I need the
> most improvement in. . . . .

If a performance standard is preferred for final assessment, we recommend each person demonstrate his/her proficiency and receive feedback on how they did.

Session One: Introduction and Orientation to Phototherapy

Goals

1. To introduce students to a theory of phototherapy.
2. To give students an introduction to the uses of phototherapy in the field.
3. To give students techniques that will allow them to begin to use phototherapy in their work settings.

Behavioral Objectives

1. Students will learn that individual perception is a relative phenomenon.
2. Students will compare perceptions of what they see and what a partner sees

when viewing the same subject matter.

3. Students will learn the basic skills in how to use a Polaroid camera by taking each other's pictures.

4. Students will discuss their own and other student's photographs, according to a set criterion, in small groups.

5. Students will share their in-class learnings in the large group.

6. Students will learn that phototherapeutic techniques can be applied in a variety of settings.

7. Students will understand that the ability to "see" a photograph is an active process of causing a figure to emerge from a ground.

8. Students will share learnings.

Class Plan

1. Photograph (instant process) each participant upon entering classroom or workshop area, have them write their names on photos and place all photos on wall or large cardboard to be available throughout workshop.

2. Introductions:
   First the instructors introduce themselves by relating to class:
   A. Who we are and how we feel about photograph (from #1)
   B. Where we work and what we do
   C. Previous phototherapy experience
   D. What brings us here now
   After instructor introductions, have participants introduce themselves by following the same procedure.

3. Overview of the course:
   A. Definition of phototherapy
   B. Four general areas of interest:
      (1) Historical, personal or family album-type photographs
      (2) Photos taken by the client of his or her world
      (3) Photos taken of client by others (including therapist)
      (4) Photos taken by client of self
   C. Class topics:
      (1) Session number one: introduction and orientation to phototherapy
      (2) Session number two: photographic self-concept and disclosure
      (3) Session number three: significance of the family album
      (4) Session number four: client photographs as projectives
      (5) Session number five: use of photo essays and photographs for closure and termination
   D. Hand out and discuss bibliography
   E. Suggested course requirements:
      (1) Students are expected to complete all assigned readings.
      (2) Students are expected to participate actively in designated

classroom work.

(3) Students are expected to bring assigned photos to class.

(4) Students are expected to maintain a notebook which shall include copies of all photos selected for class assignments.

(5) Students are expected to develop a photo essay about some aspect of their life to be brought to class and shared the last session.

4. People as cameras (exercise)

Directions: Choose a partner. Each person will take a turn as both a "camera" and a "photographer." The photographer chooses four images he/she wishes to record and maneuvers the camera into the best position to make the image. The camera keeps its eyes closed unless it is making the actual exposure, at which time the photographer taps his/her head and the camera opens its eyes and closes them immediately. This is the only time the camera's eyes are open during the exercise. Likewise, there is no talking. When the photographer has made all four photographs, both he/she and the camera separately sketch the images. You may not look at each other's photos or discuss them until the roles have been reversed and the photographic recording and subsequent sketching are completed.

In discussing the exercise, students should pay attention to their personal experience in both roles, the similarities and differences in the sketches, and if some images were easier than others to remember. The results of these discussions will be shared in the large group.

5. Lecture on phototherapy and the nature of our perception: Lecture will cover material such as that found in chapter 1, Reality photography and psychotherapy, in Dr. Krauss and J.L. Fryrear (Eds.) *Phototherapy in Mental Health.* The lecture will be mixed with class discussion concerning the material.

6. Individual portraits (exercise)

Directions: short instruction in the use of the Polaroid camera. Partners will make one photograph of each other. The subject of the photo directs the photographer as to where and how the photo will be taken. After each partner has had his/her picture taken, they will form a small group with not more than four students and do the following:

• What is something you like about this photograph? Is there anything you dislike?

• Is there anything in this photograph that you would like to change?

• If we took another photo of you in six months, what would we see different?

• In viewing this photograph,
   I see . . .
   I feel . . .

• Describe the image in one sentence.

• Caption the image.

• The photograph and the responses are to be put in a notebook.

7. Brief discussion of how we can use these techniques in our work situations, and our learnings from this session.
8. Personal data sheets are handed out, filled in, and collected.
9. Assignment:
   For next session, bring in six photographs that describe you and your world. Read the following:
   Akeret, R. Photoanalysis. New York: Peter H. Wyden, Inc., 1973.
   Gasson, A. Chapter 3, "The problem of meaning," in *Handbook for Contemporary Photography*. (4th Edition) Rochester: Light Impressions, 1977.
   Gosciewski, W. Photo counseling. *Personnel and Guidance Journal* 1975, April *53* (8), 600-604.
   Krauss, D. Reality, Photography and Psychotherapy in D. Krauss and J.L. Fryrear (Eds.), *Phototherapy in Mental Health*. Springfield, Illinois: Charles C Thomas, Publisher, 1983.
   Stewart, D. Phototherapy comes of age, *Kansas Quarterly,* 1979, *11*(4) 19-46.

Session Two: Phototherapy and Self-Concept

Goals

1. To allow students to share parts of their personal history through large and small group discussions of photos.
2. To continue building a sense of community and openness in the classroom.
3. To encourage small risk-taking behaviors in answering questions in the large and small groups.
4. To demonstrate how individual self-concepts show up in photographs.

Behavioral Objectives

1. Students will write captions for their six self-concept photographs.
2. Students will present and discuss their six photos in the small group.
3. Students will share background information on each photo.
4. Nonpresenting students will ask the presenting students questions and make observations as the photos are presented.
5. Presenting students will answer questions based on their photos in the small group.
6. Small groups will choose one photo per group to be presented in the large group.
7. Students will answer questions and make statements based on their photographs in the large group.
8. Nonpresenting students will ask presenting students questions and make observations based on the presented photos.
9. Students will discuss ways of involving clients in phototherapy.

10. Students will discuss ways of improving client self-concept via photography.
11. Students will evaluate the session in terms of what they learned/relearned/ discovered, what they wonder, and what they would like.
12. Students will share these learnings with the class.

Class Plan

1. Administrative details. Then divide into small groups (3-6) of equal size.
2. Small groups. Students will caption each of their six photos and then will, in turn, explain the choice of photo and caption to the other members. The small group's task is to draw out the presenter by asking pertinent questions based on the presenter's explanations, affect, speed, and order of presentation. The group also makes observations based on presented information. Each student will have the small group choose one of his/her photographs to be presented to the large group. The criteria used in this decision are up to the group.
3. Large group. The class meets as a whole to view and discuss selected individual photographs. These photographs are shown on a TV monitor via a video camera, deck, and monitor set-up. The large group's task is similar to that of the small group in terms of asking questions and making observations based on the presented photographs.
4. Large group discussion of larger issues for therapy, such as using client photos and discussion as a gauge of resistance and self-disclosure.
5. Assignment. The assignment for next session is to bring in six family photographs, and read the following:
   Anderson, C.M., and Malloy, E.S. Family photographs: In treatment and training. *Family Process,* 1976, *(2),* 259-264.
   Entin, A., The family photo album as icon: Photographs in family psychotherapy. In D. Krauss and J.L. Fryrear (Eds.) *Phototherapy in Mental Health.* Springfield, IL: Charles C Thomas, Publisher, 1983.
   Kaslow, F.W. and Friedman, J. Utilization of family photos and movies in family therapy. *Journal of Marriage and Family Counseling,* 1977, *3*(1), 19-25.
   Ruben, A.G. The family picture. *Journal of Marriage and Family Counseling,* 1978, *4*(3), 25-28.

Session Three: Phototherapy and Family Photographs

Goals

1. To introduce the students to some of the ways that family photographs are used in counseling and therapy.

2. To give the students some phototherapy techniques to use with families or individuals.
3. To have the instructor model techniques of working with family photographs.
4. To increase the sense of community and trust by sharing personal aspects of family photographs.

Behavioral Objectives

1. Students will view slide presentation of family photos.
2. Students will discuss the slides and their possible implications for therapy.
3. Students will present personal family photographs in small groups.
4. Students will discuss family photos in small groups.
5. Students will share background information on each photo.
6. Students will answer questions about their photographs in the small groups.
7. The nonpresenting students will ask the presenting students pertinent questions and make observations based on the photographs and their explanations.
8. Nonpresenting students will pay attention to the order in which photographs are presented, affect in the presenter, speed of presentation, and overall depth of explanation. They will ask questions and make observations based on these data.
9. Small groups will choose one photo from the group to be presented to the large group.
10. The student and his/her group will answer questions and give information about the family photograph in the large group.
11. Nonpresenting students in the large group have the same roles that they had in the small groups. They ask questions and make comments on both the content of the photograph and the process by which the photograph is shared.
12. Students will evaluate the session in terms of what they learned/relearned/discovered, what they wonder, and what they would like.
13. Students will share these learnings with the class.

Class Plan

1. Administrative details.
2. Discussion of family photos.
3. Small groups. Each student in turn presents six family photographs, introduces the family members who are portrayed, gives background information, and answers questions based on his/her presentation. The group

also asks questions and makes comments based upon the order of presentation, the affect of the presenter, speed of presentation, and overall depth of explanation.

When everyone in the group has presented his/her photos, the group chooses one photograph to be presented to the large group. The group uses its own criteria for selection of the photograph.

4. Large group. The class meets as a whole to view and discuss the individual family photographs that have been chosen by the small groups. The large group has the same task in working with these photos as they had in the small group settings; i.e. ask questions and make comments on the presented photos and the process by which they are presented.

5. Role play. A family photograph will be chosen to be acted out. Family members will be chosen from the class and briefed as to their roles. The family will be recreated or sculpted. Each member of the family in turn will create and photograph the family sculpture. The session will start by comparing the members' views of the family structure in a "family therapy" setting.

6. The role play will be processed by the class.

7. Large group discussion. What are other ways of using photographs with families?

8. Assignment. Students are to bring in six photographs that include some photos they "keep coming back to" and photographs in which "something appears to be missing to them."

Read the following:

Hammer, K. *The Clinical Application of Projective Drawing.* Springfield, Illinois: Charles C Thomas, Publisher, 1958.

Krauss, D.A. Phototherapy: Illuminating the Visual Metaphor, in D. Krauss and J.L. Fryrear (Eds.). *Phototherapy in Mental Health,* Springfield, Illinois: Charles C Thomas, Publisher, 1983.

Perls, F., Hefferline, R.F., and Goodman, P. *Gestalt Therapy.* New York: Dell Publishing, 1951, pp. 211-224.

Walker, J. The Photograph as a Catalyst in Individual Psychotherapy in Krauss and Fryrear (Eds.). *Phototherapy in Mental Health.* Springfield, Illinois: Charles C Thomas, Publisher, 1983.

White, M. Extended Perception Through Photography and Suggestion in H. Otto (Ed.) *Ways of Growth,* New York: Viking Press, 1969, pp. 34-48.

Session Four: Photographs Used as Projective Devices

Goals

1. To look at content areas of photographs as projections of our own personalities.

2. To bring into awareness areas of our personality by "owning" and working with projective aspects of photographs.
3. To model a therapy session that uses the projective aspects of photos as primary stimulus.

Behavioral Objectives

1. Students will relearn that perception is a relative phenomenon.
2. Students will bring to class and discuss personal projective photographs.
3. Students will make photographs during the class and discuss them as parts of themselves.
4. Students will discuss the concept of projection.
5. Students will observe a phototherapy session where projective use of photos is the primary stimulus.
6. Students will make observations about the session in the large group.
7. Students will ask questions based on the session in the large group.

Class Plan

1. Administrative details.
2. Small groups. Small groups equipped with Polaroid camera, film, and flash cubes will make two or three photos per person in the classroom, the building, or around the immediate grounds. The task is to "make two or three photographs of things that interest you and/or become foreground in your environment."

   When students return to the classroom, each student captions his/her photographs and selects one image to write a paragraph about. In writing, students are asked to "own the images"; i.e. writes in "I" language as though the image could speak. Some of these photos and writings are shared with the class.
3. Discussion. What do these photos and stories communicate about ourselves? What other ideas do you have as effective means to use photos in a projective manner?
4. Large group. Discussion of projection and the various orientations toward it. Projection in the Freudian model and the Gestalt model, projection as a way to make sense out of the world, and the differences between unaware and aware projection will be discussed.
5. Relaxation exercise. Class will participate in a relaxation exercises as a way of warming up to begin a phototherapy session in which the photograph is used projectively as the primary stimulus in the session.
6. Phototherapy demonstration session. Session will use a student and his/her photograph to demonstrate techniques of using photographs projectively.
7. Processing the session. The class will share feelings, questions, and com-

ments as a result of observing the session.
8. Assignment: Read the following and bring your own photo essay:
Jury, M. and Jury, D. *Gramp.* New York: Penguin Books, 1978.
Kübler-Ross, E. and Warshaw, M. *To Live Until We Say Goodbye.* Englewood Cliffs, New Jersey: Prentice-Hall, 1978.
Mikler, M.E., Using photographs in the termination phase. *Social Work,* 1977, 22(4), 318-319.
Richards, E. Dorries Journey, *American Photographer,* 6(6), June 1981, 48-61.

Session Five: Approaches to the Photo Essay and Uses of Photos in Termination, Separation, and Grief Work

Goals

1. To demonstrate approaches and effectiveness of the photo essay.
2. To demonstrate approaches and effectiveness of photographs used for issues of termination, separation, and grief work.
3. To summarize course work.
4. To provide a sense of closure and termination for the course.
5. To get evaluation and feedback from students on the sequence and content of the workshop.

Behavioral Objectives

1. Students will learn various ways to construct photo essays with their clients.
2. Students will see examples of some approaches to photo essay work.
3. Students will hear, see, and discuss how photographs may be used in working on issues in termination, separation, and grief work.
4. Students will generate a list of topic areas, assignments, projects, and exercises that were included in this course.
5. Students will evaluate the class in terms of what they learned/relearned/ discovered, what they wonder, and what they would like.
6. Students will evaluate the training workshop as a whole in terms of topic areas, exercises, assignments, and their individual experiences.

Class Plan

1. Administrative details.
2. Lecture on creating of photo essays. Areas include:
(a) asking clients to put together some of their personal photographs with a set order and captions; (b) a "life up till now" book which is an illustrated

autobiography; (c) collage made from magazine pictures which illustrate important objects or values in a client's life; (d) a collection of self-pictures: social self, private self, happy self, zany self, spiritual self, etc.; (e) asking clients to compose a story from candids that the therapist has taken of the client over time in different social situations; (f) giving the client a number of fairly undifferentiated or "projective" photographs and asking him/her to compose a story; (g) using animation or video tape in this process.

Class Plan

3. Small group discussion of our photo essays. Group members are to listen to presenter, ask questions and give feedback regarding the individual photo essays. Themes of the essay may be briefly explored with its presenter.
4. In a large group setting, class members share their essays, discuss the themes and their learnings from this assignment. Class members are encouraged to ask questions and give feedback.
5. Class-generated course summary. Areas or topics covered, assignments, exercises, projects, and their individual experiences.
6. Lecture, demonstration, and discussion around the use of photos in termination, separation, and grief work.
7. Class evaluation and feedback in terms of what they learned/relearned/discovered, what they wonder, and what they would like to know more about.
8. Course evaluation and feedback in terms of topic areas, assignments, exercises, projects, and individual experiences.

Summary and Conclusions

People in our society are ready for the incorporation of photographs and the photographic process in their therapeutic relationships. The availability of photo biographical data combined with the simplicity of obtaining here and now photographs during therapy, makes phototherapy an easy adjunctive technique to learn and apply in therapy. The idea of Hugh Diamond in the 1850s of applying photography in the clinical setting can now be accomplished with ease.

As mentioned in the first part of this chapter, research conducted by the authors has demonstrated that the concepts and methods presented in this chapter can be taught and learned by mental health practitioners. A quasi-experimental research project using pre- and post-testing and self-report questions revealed some interesting and supportive results. A by-product of this training, as reported by participants, is their own personal development and professional integration. When compared with a control class (an alternative treatment group completing graduate degrees in counseling), the phototherapy students demonstrated significantly greater ability to focus on the content of photographs in a therapeutic manner. Phototherapy students were able to ask more pertinent therapeutic questions, and make more therapeutic comments about client photographs, make more astute observations about the photographic data, utilize more "process" inquiry (as compared to content inquiry), and were also able to better adapt pre-existing counseling skills into the phototherapeutic experience than the control group.

Further analysis of selected variables on the phototherapy (experimental) and counseling (control) students revealed no pre- or post-test changes for the control group. As a matter of fact, an interesting finding was that the control group scored higher than the phototherapy class on most items (questions and comments about client photos) on the pretest. Our correlational analysis revealed "no" correlations between responses on test items and interest in photography, age, sex, or counseling experience of students.

In conclusion, we have demonstrated through various teaching/learning approaches, such as the one described in this chapter, that phototherapy methods and theory can be readily learned by mental health professionals and that these learnings form a logical fit with existing therapeutic skills. Phototherapy has been shown to be an effective, programmatic and potent therapeutic process which is readily available and incorporable into one's professional repertoire.

Summary

JERRY L. FRYREAR AND DAVID A. KRAUSS

T HE use of photography in therapy has a history almost as old as that of photography itself. In 1856, Dr. Hugh Diamond presented the first known paper on this subject to the Royal Society of Medicine in England. His presentation advanced the theory of using photography as part of the practice of psychiatry. He suggested that photographs could be used to study the appearance of the mentally ill, that photographs could be used in the treatment of mentally ill by using portraits to effect self-concept changes, and that photographs could be used to record faces, which would be a useful tool for later record keeping concerning treatment and/or readmission.

The use of phototherapeutic techniques has continued and expanded in the helping professions, but in a relatively isolated manner. Reports of photo counseling, photoanalysis, and phototherapy have appeared from time to time in the psychotherapy literature, and workers who have used these techniques have by and large been unaware of other workers with similar interests. Very recently, phototherapy has emerged as a distinct entity, with a coherent network of phototherapy workers and a growing body of literature.

Phototherapy is an eclectic approach to psychotherapy and embraces a broad spectrum of techniques. It may be practiced in ways that are consistent with the psychoanalytic, behavioral and/or humanistic schools of psychology. In this book we have presented original essays by contemporary workers who use photography in a surprising variety of ways and from disparate but not contradictory points of view.

One pervasive point of view is that people are not only verbal and able to process language symbols, but they are also visual and able to process images in meaningful ways quite apart from whatever written or verbal explanations accompany them. That point of view is germane to any of the approaches described in this book. The approaches differ in the choice of images to use in the therapy, and the particular manner in which the images are incorporated into the treatment program. Photographs of the client, photographs by the client, abstract photos, and family album photos are all used in therapeutic ways.

We began this book by reviewing the phototherapy literature and concluded that the reports could be divided into twelve broad areas. They are (1) using photographic images to evoke certain emotional states; (2) using photography to elicit verbal behavior; (3) using photographs of others as models; (4) teaching photography as a skill; (5) using photography to facilitate socialization; (6) using photography as a form of creative expression; (7) using photographs as a diagnostic adjunct to verbal therapy; (8) using photography as a form of nonverbal communication between client and therapist; (9) using photographs of or by the client to document change; (10) using photographs to prolong certain experiences; (11) using photographs of the client as self-confrontation; and (12) training therapists to use photography as therapy.

In the chapters that followed the authors presented work that covered most of the twelve areas just mentioned. Douglas Stewart set phototherapy in historical context in Chapter 2, by reviewing the history of photography and pointing out how this medium lends itself particularly well to therapy, for both technical and social reasons. Technically, the medium is extremely simple, or can be, and the photograph is available within minutes. Socially, the photograph, particularly the "snapshot," has come to be the visual history of our culture, and on a personal level, the objects or other people photographed somehow become part of the photographer's identity and personal domain.

Following Stewart's historical overview, David A. Krauss addressed the relationship among reality, photography and psychotherapy in Chapter 3. Krauss maintains that photographs represent a metaphoric map that relates to one's participation in life. Phototherapy, as a psychotherapy approach, allows clients to examine their lives and to review their personal histories through the use of snapshots and the family album. It also encourages clients to communicate visually how they experience the world, and to discover the important personal symbols they choose to express that experience.

In Chapter 4, Krauss further developed the premise of the visual metaphor. He discussed the pictorial nature of the metaphor and the use of visually referent language and photography as a potent combination in therapy.

Chapter 5 was devoted to a discussion of a somewhat different rationale for phototherapy, that of visual self-confrontation. In that chapter, Jerry L. Fryrear discussed the concepts of self-concept, self-esteem, and self-confrontation and gave examples of the use of photographs of the client to enhance self-esteem by confronting the conceptualizing and esteeming process that the client is applying to himself or herself.

Robert Ziller and his colleagues discussed, in Chapter 6, photographs *by* clients as they revealed the "psychological niche" each client perceived for herself or himself. In Krauss's words, the "photographic self-concepts" thus revealed represent a visual metaphor for the client's participation in life.

In Chapter 7, Alan D. Entin illustrated the use of photographs in family therapy. He particularly attempted to explain how photographs from the family album could fit into Bowen's family system theory, and discussed the systems concepts of triangulation, differentiation, and emotional cut off. Family photographs and family albums are a rich source of information about family relationships, for both therapist and client.

Ambiguous visual stimuli have been used for years as projective techniques for diagnostic purposes. Joel Walker, in Chapter 8, described the therapeutic use of ambiguous visual stimuli — photographs that he had taken and found to be useful with his clients. Much of Walker's discussion is from a psychoanalytic point of view, as he demonstrated how photographs could be used to explore transferential feelings, work through conflicts, and deal with resistance to therapy.

Robert I. Wolf, in Chapter 9, also discussed phototherapy within a psychoanalytic context. His work combines photography and other visual art in working with children and adolescents. His use of instant photography provides the clients with immediate gratification, and the clients then embellish the photographs in a variety of ways with other visual media such as paints or cray-pas. Wolf likens the playful aspect of his work to the traditional free association of verbal psychoanalysis.

From a humanistic perspective, Judy Weiser works with people who are "different." Her phototherapy was described in Chapter 10. Because of the extreme difficulties of using verbal approaches with people who are handicapped, such as deaf children, or people from different cultures, Weiser has found photography to be an indispensible tool with her clients.

Lest phototherapy be thought of as a "fad" or a therapeutic tool without any real integration into the overall field of psychotherapy, Brian Zakem gave a brief outline of a system of phototherapy within the broader framework of mental health. That outline was offered as Chapter 11. Zakem gave an example of a clinical application of the system within a community mental health center.

We concluded the book with a description of a training program for phototherapists. That chapter was written by David A. Krauss and Ansel L. Woldt, who have had a great deal of experience with such training. They describe exercises, offer a bibliography, and outline a curriculum, all of which should be of great interest to people wanting to learn the elements of phototherapy.

There is no doubt that phototherapy is a viable treatment modality. There is also little doubt that its use will continue to expand and continue to be refined. There is now an International Phototherapy Association, and several centers and institutes for the expansion and refinement of phototherapeutic theory and practice. The International Phototherapy Association publishes case studies, research reports, theoretical essays, and other information in *Phototherapy*, which keeps members and subscribers informed about the field. There is also a related organization called Video Researchers in Psychology whose members are interested in the application of video technology to psychological problems. In other fields there are the journals *Visual Sociology,*

Visual Communication (in anthropology) and *The Arts in Psychotherapy*. There is also the International Visual Literacy Association, which is broadly interested in visual learning.

With the current communication among phototherapy adherents and the high level of professionalism and interest shown, it seems likely that phototherapy in mental health will continue to thrive and achieve even highter levels of sophistication.

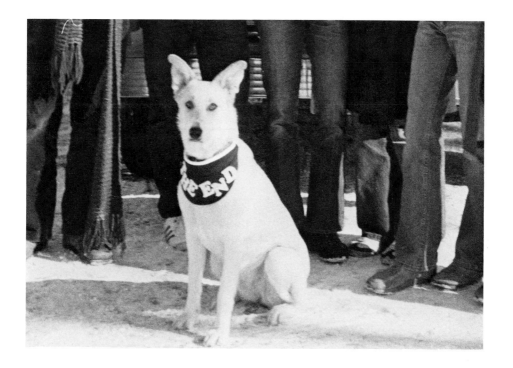

Photo by David A. Krauss

Appendix

Selected Phototherapy References

Akeret, R.V. *Photoanalysis.* New York: Peter H. Wyden, Inc., 1973.

Ammerman, M.S., & Fryrear, J.L. Photographic enhancement of children's self esteem. *Psychology in the Schools,* 1975, *12*(3), 319-325.

Anderson, C.M., & Malloy, E.S. Family photographs: In treatment and training. *Family Process,* 1976, *15*(2), 259-264.

Arieti, S. *Creativity: The magic synthesis.* New York: Basic Books, 1976.

Arnheim, R. *Art and visual perception* (new version). Berkeley: University of California Press, 1974.

Arnheim, R. On the nature of photography. *Critical Inquiry,* 1974, *1,* 149-161.

Arnheim, R. *Visual thinking.* Berkeley: University of California Press, 1971.

Becker, H. Photography and sociology. *Studies in the Anthropology of Visual Communication,* 1974, *5,* 3-26.

Bloomer, C.M. *Principles of visual perception.* New York: Van Nostrand Reinhold, 1976.

Brown, G. *Human teaching for human learning:* An introduction to confluent education. New York: Viking Press, 1971.

Brown, G., editor, with Yeomans, T., & Grizzand, L. (Ed.) *The live classroom: Innovation through confluent education and gestalt.* New York, Viking Press, 1975.

Byers, P. Cameras don't take pictures. *Columbia University Forum,* 1966, *9*(1), 27-32.

Byers, P. Still photography in the systematic recording and anaylsis of behavioral data. *Human Organization,* 1964, *23,* 78-84.

Chalfen, R. Photoanalysis. *Studies in the Anthropology of Visual Communication,* 1974, *5,*57-59.

Cloniger, S.J. The sexually dimorphic image: An empirical analysis of the influences of gender differences on photographic content (Doctoral dissertation, The Ohio State University, 1975). *Dissertation Abstracts International,* 1975, *35,* 8-A. (University Microfilms No. 5527)

Coblentz, A.L. Use of photographs in a family mental health clinic. *American Journal of Psychiatry,* 1964, *121,* 601-602.

Combs, J.M., & Ziller, R.C. Photographic self-concept of counselees. *Journal of Counseling Psychology,* 1977, *24*(7), 452-455.

Cornelison, F.S., & Arsenian, J. A study of the response of psychotic patients to photographic self-image experience. *Psychiatric Quarterly,* 1960, *34*(1), 1-8.

Diamond, H. On the application of photography to the physiognomic and mental phenomena of insanita. In S. Gilman (Ed.), *The face of madness.* New York: Brunner/Mazel, 1976.

Entin, A.D. Photo therapy: Family albums and multigenerational portraits. *Camera Lucida,* 1980, *1*(2), 39-51.

Entin, A.D. The use of photography in family psychotherapy. Paper presented to the American Psychological Association Convention, 1979.

Entin, A.D. Reflection of families. *Phototherapy Quarterly* 2(2), September 1979, 19-21.

Ekman, P. Face muscles talk every language. *Psychology Today,* 1975, 9(4).

Fox, C. and Wortman, C.B. A therapeutic use of film. *American Journal of Art Therapy,* 1975, 15,

229

19-21.

Fryrear, J.L. A selective non-evaluation review of research on phototherapy. *Phototherapy Quarterly* 2(3), April 1980, 7-9.

Fryrear, J.L., Nuell, L.R., & Ridley, S.D. Photographic self-concept enhancement of male juvenile delinquents. *Journal of Consulting and Clinical Psychology,* 1974, 42(6), 915.

Fryrear, J.L., Nuell, L.R., & White, P. Enhancement of male juvenile delinquents' self concepts through photographed social interactions. *Journal of Clinical Psychology,* 1977, 33(3), 833-838.

Garner, G. A psychologist observes photography: An interview of Dr. Stanley Milgram. *Camera 35,* 1977.

Gass, W.H. On photography (a book review). *New York Times Book Review,* Dec, 18, 1977, 7 and 30.

Gasson, A. The documentary dilemma. *Kansas Quarterly,* 1979, 11(4), 125-130.

Gasson, A. *A chronology of photography.* Athens, Ohio, Handbook Co., 1972.

Gasson, A. *Handbook for contemporary photography* (4th Edition) Rochester: Light Impressions, 1977.

Gasswint, C.D. Changes in self-concept as a function of immediate self-image confrontation (Doctoral dissertation, University of Oklahoma, 1968). *Dissertation Abstracts International,* 1968, *29.* (University Microfilms No. 1839-B)

Gellert, E., Girgus, J.S., & Cohen, J. Children's awareness of their bodily appearance: A developmental study of factors associated with the body percept. *Genetic Psychology Monographs,* 1971, *84*(1), 109-174.

Gill, N.T. The relationship between modes of perception and selected variables in young children (Doctoral dissertation, University of Florida, 1965). *Dissertation Abstracts International,* 1965, *27.* (University Microfilms No. 673-A)

Gill, N.T., & Messina, R. Visual self-confrontation and the self-concept of the exceptional child. *Florida Journal of Educational Research,* 1973, *15,* 18-36.

Gilman, S. (Ed.). *The face of madness.* New York: Brunner/Mazel, 1976.

Gombrich, E.H. The visual image. *Scientific American,* 1972, *227*(3), 82-96.

Gosciewski, W.F. Photo counseling. *Personnel and Guidance Journal,* 1975, *53*(8), 600-604.

Graham, J.R. The use of photographs in psychiatry. *Canadian Psychiatric Association Journal,* 1967, *12,* 425.

Green, J. (Ed.). *The snapshot.* Millerton, N.Y.: Aperture, Inc., 1974.

Gregory, R.L. *Eye and brain: the psychology of seeing.* New York: World University Library, 1966.

Gunther, Thomas K. Photo groups in German prison for women. Presented at International Photo Therapy Symposium. DeKalb, Illinois, May 1979.

Hall, D.G. Photography as a learning experience in self-perception. (Doctoral Dissertation, University of Michigan, 1980).

Hall, J.B., Biographical essay. In M. Hoffman (Ed.), *Minor White: Rites and passages.* Millerton, N.Y.: Aperture, Inc., 1978.

Hattersley, R. 30 ways photography is good for you, *Popular Photography*, 86(2), February, 1980 87-127.

Hattersley, R. *Discover yourself through photography.* New York: Morgan and Morgan, 1971.

Hedges, R.E. Photography and self-concept. *Audiovisual Instruction,* 1972, *17*(5), 26-28.

Hedges, R., Nicoletti, D., & Tyding, K. *Self-directed children's photography.* New York: Photo-Lix, Inc., 1972.

Hoffman, M. (Ed.), *Minor White: Rites and passages.* Millerton, N.Y.: Aperture, Inc., 1978.

Holzman, P.S., On hearing and seeing oneself. *Journal of Nervous and Mental Disease,* 1969, *148*(3), 198-209.

Jaffe, D.J., & Bressler, D.E. The use of guided imagery as an adjunct to medical diagnosis and treatment. *Journal of Humanistic Psychology,* 1980, 20(4), 47-59.

Kaslow, F.W., & Friedman, J. Utilization of family photos and movies in family therapy. *Journal of Marriage and Family Counseling,* 1977, *3*(1), 19-25.

Kaslow, F. What personal photos reveal about marital sex conflicts. *Journal of Marital and Sex Therapy,* 1979, *5*(2), 134-141.

Kotkin, A. The family album as a form of folklore. *Exposure,* 1978, *16*(1), 4-8.

Korzybski, A. *Science and sanity,* New York: International Non-Aristotelian Library Publishing Co., 1933.

Krauss, D. A summary of characteristics of photographs which make them useful in counseling and therapy. *Camera Lucida,* 1980, *1*(2), 2-12.

Krauss, D. Photography, imaging, and visually referent language in therapy: Illuminating the metaphor. *Camera Lucida,* 1982, 5.

Krauss, D. The uses of still photography in counseling and therapy: development of a training model. (Doctoral dissertation, Kent State University, 1979.)

Krauss, D. The uses of still photography in counseling and therapy: Development of a training model (illustrated dissertation abstract). *Photo Therapy Quarterly* 2(3), 12-13.

Krauss, D., Utilyzing photographs and visual language in therapy: Illuminating the metaphor, *Photo Therapy,* 1981, *2*(4), 6-7.

Kubler-Ross, E., & Warshaw, M. *To live until we say goodbye.* Englewood Cliffs, New Jersey: Prentice-Hall, 1978.

Kulich, R.J., & Goldberg, R.W. Differences in the production of photographs: a potential assessment technique. *Perceptual and Motor Skills,* 1978, *47,* 223-229.

Langsan, N., Levinson, R., & Teller, A. *Photography in the classroom: a workbook.* Chicago: Illinois Arts Council, 1975.

Lesy, M., *Time Frames: The meaning of family pictures.* New York: Pantheon Books, 1980.

Lesy, M., Snapshots: Psychological documents, frozen dreams. *Afterimage,* Rochester, N.Y., 1976, *4*(4), 12-13.

Levison, R. Psychodynamically oriented Photo Therapy. *Photo Therapy Quarterly,* *2*(2), Sept. 1979, 14-16.

Lewis, M.E., & Butler, R.N. Life review therapy. *Geriatrics,* Nov., 1974, 165-173.

Lindley, D.A. Photography and the way of self. *Kansas Quarterly,* 1979, *11*(4), 11-17.

Loellbach, M. Case illustration, *Photo therapy quarterly,* 1978, *1*(3), 2-3.

Loellbach, M. The uses of photographic materials in psychotherapy: A literature review. Unpublished master's thesis, George Williams College, 1978.

McDougall-Treacy, G. The person as camera experience. *Photo Therapy Quarterly,* *2*(2), Sept., 1979, 16-18.

McKinney, J.P. Photo counseling. *Children Today,* 1979, *8*(1), 29.

Meiselas, S. *Learn to see: A sourcebook of photography projects by teachers and students.* Cambridge, Mass.: Polaroid Corporation, 1974.

Metz, G. Perception and photography. *Camera Lucida,* 1981, *1*(3), 5-19.

Milgram, S. The image freezing machine. *Psychology Today,* January 1977, pp. 50-54; 108.

Miller, M.F. Responses of psychiatric patients to their photographed images. *Diseases of the Nervous System,* 1962, *23,* 296-298.

Muse, K. Photo one: *Basic photo text.* Englewood Cliffs, New Jersey: Prentice-Hall, 1972.

Musello, C. Context, Structure and "photographic behavior:" the studio portrait session. *Studies in Visual Communication* (in press 1982)

Musello, C. Family photography: In J. Wagner (ed.), *Images of information.* Beverly Hills, CA: Sage, 1979.

Musello, C. Studying the home mode: an exploration of family photography and visual communication. *Studies in Visual Communication.* 1980, *6*(1), 24-41.

Muhl, A.M. Notes on the use of photography in checking up unconscious conflicts. *Psychoanalytic Review,* 1927, *14,* 329-331.

Myers, E.S. Photographic images as a visual induction into an alpha and/or altered state of consciousness (Doctoral dissertation, Boston University, 1977). *Dissertation Abstracts International,* 1977, 38(4-A), 2005-A.

Nathan, D.J. The use of self confrontation through photography or videotape as a therapeutic method for changing self image and aiding weight maintenance in formerly obese adults (Doctoral dissertation, University of Miami, 1978). Dissertation Abstracts International, 1978, *39*(11), 6659-A.

Nelson-Gee, E. Learning to be: A look into the use of therapy with Polaroid photography as a means of recreating the development of perception and the ego. *Art Psychotherapy,* 1975, *2*(2), 159-164.

Nicoletti, D.J. An investigation into the effects of a self-directed photography experience upon the self-concept of fourth grade students. (Doctoral dissertation, Syracuse University, 1972). *Dissertation Abstracts International,* 1972, *32*, 11-A. (University Microfilms No. 6213)

Passikoff, R.K. Student attention as measured by photoanalysis and kind of instruction as predictors of achievement (Doctoral Dissertation New York University 1977) *Dissertation Abstracts International,* 1977, *38*, 2-A, 750-751.

Perls, F., Hefferline, R.F., & Goodman, P. *Gestalt therapy,* New York: Dell Publishing, 1951.

Polster, E., & Polster, M. *Gestalt therapy integrated.* New York: Vintage Books, Random House, 1973.

Reusch, J. *Nonverbal communication.* Berkeley: University of California Press, 1969.

Robbins, A., & Sibley, L.B. *Creative art therapy.* New York: Brunner/Mazel, Inc., 1976.

Robbins, L.L. Photography. *Bulletin of the Menninger Clinic,* 1942, *6*(3), 89-91.

Ruben, A.G. The family picture. *Journal of Marriage and Family Counseling,* 1978, *4*(3), 25-28.

Ruby, J. In a pic's eye: Interpretive strategies for deriving significance and meaning from photographs. *Afterimage 3*(9), 5-7.

Ruby, J. Seeing through pictures: the anthropology of photography. *Camera Lucida,* 1981, *1*(3), 20-33.

Sackeim, H.A., Gur, R.C., & Saucy, M.C. Emotions are expressed more intensely on the left side of the face. *Science,* 1978(Act) *202,* 434-436.

Sampson, P.H.; Ray, T.S.; Pugh, L.A., & Clark, M.L. Picture recognition as an index of social sensitivity in chronic schizophrenia: the effects of chlorpromazine. *Journal of Consulting Psychology,* 1962, *26*(6), 510-514.

Samuels, M., & Samuels, N. *Seeing with the mind's eye.* New York: Random House, 1975.

Scheflin, A.E. *Body language and social order: Communication as behavioral control.* Englewood Cliffs, New Jersey: Prentice-Hall, 1972.

Schutz, W. *Joy: Expanding human awareness.* New York: Grove Press, 1967.

Segall, M.H., Campbell, D.T., & Herskovitz, M.J. *The influence of culture on visual perception.* Indianapolis: Bobbs-Merrill, 1966.

Sekula, A. On the invention of meaning in photographs. *Artforum,* 1975, *13*(5), 36-45.

Seskin, M. Photobiography: A phenomenologically based approach to human story and personal insight (Doctoral dissertation, Calif. School of Prof. Psych., 1978). *Dissertation Abstracts International,* 1978, *38*, 9-B. (University Microfilms No. 4481-B)

Smith, J.R. Taking portrait photographs of children in therapy. *Photo Therapy Quarterly,* 1978, *1*(4), 1-2.

Sontag, S. *On photography.* New York: Farrar, Strauss and Giroux, 1977.

Spire, R.H. Photographic self-image confrontation. *American Journal of Nursing,* 1973, *73*(7), 1207-1210.

Stewart, D. Photo therapy: Theory and practice. *Art Psychotherapy,* 1979, *6*(1), 41-46.

Stewart, D. *Photography and psychology join hands.* Northern Illinois University, 1978 (Unpublished paper.)

Stewart, D. Photo Therapy and Contemporary therapy theories — Gestalt Therapy, *Photo Therapy Quarterly,* *2*(1), 1979, 16-18.

Stewart, D. The uses of photo therapy in self-image change. Unpublished paper. 1979.

Stewart, D. Photo therapy comes of age, *Kansas Quarterly,* 1979, *11*(4), 19-46.

Sturr, E. (Ed.) (entire issue on "Photography and contemporary society"). *Kansas Quarterly,* 1979, *11*(4).

Sulzberger, C.F. Unconscious motivations of the amateur photographer. *Psychoanalysis,* 1955, *3* (3), 18-24.

Swedlung, C. *Photography: A handbook of history, materials and processes.* New York: Holt, Rinehart and Winston, 1974.

Szarkowski, J. *The photographer's eye.* New York Graphic Society, Boston, 1966.

Szarkowski, J. *Looking at photographs.* New York: Rappaport Printing Corp., 1973.

Tamashiro, R.T. Using photography to amplify self-esteem in the primary grades. *Educational Perspectives,* 1971, *10,* 7-12.

Teller, A. Some questions for photo therapy. *Photo Therapy Quarterly,* 1979, *2*(2), 12-13.

Teller, A., Langsan, N., & Levinson, R. *Photography in the classroom: A workbook.* Springfield: Illinois Arts Council, 1975.

Thelen, H. *Education and the human quest.* New York: Harper and Row, 1960.

Titus, S.L. Family photographs and the transition to parenthood. *Journal of Marriage and the Family,* 1976, *38*(3), 525-530.

Trusso, J. Some uses of instant photography in holistic therapy. *Photo Therapy Quarterly,* 1979, *2*(1), 14-15.

Turner, P., Photographs, demands and expectations. In J. Bayer (Ed.), *Reading photographs.* New York: Pantheon Books, 1977, 77-80.

Turner-Hogan, P. The use of group photo therapy in the classroom. *Photo Therapy,* 1981, *2*(4), 13.

Turner-Hogan, P. The use of photography as a social work technique. Unpublished paper, San Jose State U., 1980.

Tyding, K. Instamatic therapy. *Human Behavior,* 1973, Feb., 30.

Ulman, E., & Dachinger, P. *Art therapy in theory and practice.* New York: Schocken Books, 1975.

Van Vliet. K. Creativity and self-image: an odyssey into poetry through photography. *Art Psychotherapy,* 1977, *4,* 88-93.

Vitales, M.S., & Smith, R.K. The prediction of vocational aptitude and success from photographs. *Journal of Experimental Psychology,* 1932, *15,* 615-629.

Vogel, R.K. The effects of an audiovisual relaxation training program upon pulse rate, skin temperature and anxiety. (Doctoral dissertation, Boston College, 1977) *Dissertation Abstracts International,* 1977, *33*(3-A), 1312.

Voss, S.H. The use of photography to study children's perceptions of themselves and others (Doctoral dissertation, University of Florida, 1968). *Dissertation Abstracts International,* 1968, *29,* 3-A. (University Microfilms No. 822)

Wagner, J. (Ed.) *Images of information: Photography and social science research,* Beverly Hills: Sage, 1979.

Walker, J.L. The photograph as a catalyst in psychotherapy. *Canadian Journal of Psychiatry,* October, 1982.

Walker, J.L. See and Tell: Audience Reactions to a Participatory Photographic Exhibition, 1979 (unpublished paper).

Walker, J.L. See and Tell: Comparative Survey, Mexico and New York, 1981 (unpublished paper).

Walker, J.L. See and Tell: A Photographic Exhibit as Therapy, 1982 (unpublished paper).

Walker, J.L. See and Tell: *Photo Therapy Quarterly,* 1980, *2*(3), 14-15.

Weal, E. Photo psychology. *Innovations,* 1980, *6*(3), 13-15.

Weiser, J. Phototherapy: photography as a verb. *The B.C. Photographer,* Fall, 1975, 33-36.

Weiss, R., & Enter, S. *Creating environments and personal awareness through the use of Polaroid camera.* Unpublished paper, Bronx-Lebanon Hospital, New York, 1975.

White, M. Equivalence: The perennial trend. In N. Lyons (Ed.), *Photographers on photography.*

Englewood Cliffs, New Jersey: Prentice-Hall Inc., 1966.

White, M. Extended perception through photography and suggestion. In H. Otto & J. Mann (Eds.), *Ways of growth.* New York: Viking Press, 1969.

White, M. Varieties of responses to photographs. *Aperture,* 1962, *10*(3), 116-128.

White, M. What is meant by "reading" photographs. *Aperture,* 1957, *5*(2), 48-50.

Wikler, M.E. Using photographs in the termination phase. *Social Work,* 1977, *22,*(4), 318-319.

Williams, R.D., & Williams, R.C.M. Photography as a bridge between institution and community: A preventive intervention. *Photo Therapy* 1981, *2*(4), 8-12.

Wolf, R. The use of instant photography in the establishment of a therapeutic alliance. Convention program, American Art Therapy Association, 1978, 20-22.

Wolf, R. The use of instant photography in creative expressive therapy: an integrative case study. *Art Psychotherapy,* 1978, *5,* 81-91.

Wolf, R. The Polaroid technique: Spontaneous dialogues from the unconscious. *Art Psychotherapy,* 1976, *3*(3/4), 197-201.

Wolz, C. Equivalent: Window or mirror. *Camera Lucida, 1*(1), 13-18.

Worthington, E.L., & Shumate, M. Imagery and verbal counseling methods in stress inoculation training for pain control. *Journal of Counseling Psychology,* 1981, *28*(1), 1-6.

Zakem, B. Photographs help patients focus on their problems (in "Newsline"). *Psychology Today,* 1977, *11*(4), 22.

Zakem, B., Kunka, J., & Cardone, L. Exploratory analysis of the uses of the TAT and personal photo photography pilot project. Unpublished paper. Ravenswood Hospital, Chicago, Illinois, 1977.

Zakem, B. *Photo therapy: A developing psychotherapeutic approach.* Unpublished paper, Ravenswood Community Mental Health Center, Chicago, Illinois, 1978.

Zakia, R. *Perception and photography.* Englewood Cliffs, New Jersey: Prentice-Hall, 1975.

Zakia, R.D. Spaced-out. *Exposure, 15*:1, 36-38.

Ziller, R.C. Psychology and photography. *The Photographer,* 1975, *2,* 7.

Ziller, R.C., & Smith, R.A. A phenomenological utilization of photographs. *Journal of Phenomenological Psychology,* 1977, *7*(2), 172-182.

Zinker, J. *Creative process in gestalt therapy.* New York: Brunner/Mazel, 1977.

Zinker, J. Dream work as theatre: An innovation in gestalt therapy. *Voices,* 1971, *7*(2), 17-25.

Zwick, D. Photography as a tool toward increased awareness of the aging self. *Art Psychotherapy,* 1978, *5,* 135-141.

Zwick, D. Photo therapy as an adjunct to group process. *Photo Therapy,* 1981, *2*(4), 3-5.

NAME INDEX

A

Abt, L., 132
Adair, J., 99, 115
Akeret, R.V., 4, 5, 8, 10, 15, 16, 21, 217, 229
Alinder, J., 131
Americkaner, N., 111, 113
Ammerman, M.S., 6, 9, 21, 77, 80, 91, 229
Amon, A.H., 13, 22
Anderson, C.M., 11, 21, 218, 229
Arbus, D., 28, 29, 38
Arieti, S., 229
Aristotle, 98
Arnheim, R., 35, 37, 38, 68, 229
Arsenian, J., 4, 18-19, 21, 75, 77-78, 92, 229

B

Bandler, R., 61, 68, 181, 199
Bandura, A., 113
Barnardo, 29
Barrow, T.F., 118, 131
Bartlett, F.C., 97, 113
Bateson, G., 61, 68
Bayer, J., 233
Becker, H., 229
Bellocq, E.J., 39
Berenson, B., 36, 38
Berger, M.M., 85, 92, 201, 208
Bergin, A., 208, 209
Berkowitz, L., 92
Billou, R.M., 98
Billow, R.M., 114
Bloomer, C.M., 229
Bogen, 36
Bowen, M., 118-119, 131
Bressler, D.E., 4, 21, 60, 230
Brown, G., 213, 229
Bugental, J.F.T., 99, 114
Bunnell, P., 31, 38
Burwen, L.S., 12, 21
Butler, R.N., 5, 17, 22, 231,
Byers, P., 38, 229

C

Camacho de Santoya, C., 14, 23

A

Campbell, D., 12, 21, 68, 232
Cardone, L., 234
Carter, E., 132
Chalfen, R., 229
Chinn, P.C., 178, 179, 199
Clark, M.L., 232
Cloniger, S.J., 229
Coblentz, A.L., 11, 21, 229
Cohen, B.D., 12-13, 21
Cohen, J., 230
Combs, J., 14, 21, 99, 100, 114, 229
Cooper, T., 38
Cornelison, F.S., 4, 18-19, 21, 75, 77-78, 92, 229
Corsini, R., 202, 209
Crane, M., 122, 131
Craven, G.M., 26, 27, 30, 33, 34-35, 38
Creighton, 60

D

Dachinger, P., 233
Daguerre, L.,25, 27, 34
Danet, B.B., 74, 92
De Lappa, W., 117, 131
Deri, S., 159, 172
Diamond, H., 3, 26, 29, 135, 201, 223, 225, 229
Disderi, 26
Dowbenko, G., 205, 209
Duval, S., 89, 92

E

Eastman, G., 31, 32
Ekman, P., 229
Elliott, G.P., 34, 38
Enter, S., 233
Entin, A.D., 5, 15, 20, 21, 74, 118, 119, 120, 121, 127, 128, 131, 132, 229
Entin, E.S., 118, 132
Esterson, A., 59-60

F

Falzett, W., 66
Fenjves, P.F., 118, 132
Fitts, W.H., 72-73, 92
Fleshman, B., 21, 85, 92, 209

235

SUBJECT INDEX